Spiritual Caregiving

Spiritual Caregiving
Healthcare as a Ministry

Verna Benner Carson and
Harold G. Koenig

Templeton Foundation Press
Philadelphia and London

Templeton Foundation Press
Five Radnor Corporate Center, Suite 120
100 Matsonford Road
Radnor, Pennsylvania 19087
www.templetonpress.org
Templeton Foundation Press helps intellectual leaders and others learn about science research on aspects of realities, invisible and intangible. Spiritual realities include unlimited love, accelerating creativity, worship, and the benefits of purpose in persons and in the cosmos.

Designed and typeset by Kachergis Book Design
Printed by Versa Press, Inc.

LIBRARY OF CONGRESS CATALOGING-IN-PUBLICATION DATA
Carson, Verna Benner.
  Spiritual Caregiving : healthcare as a ministry / Verna Benner Carson and Harold G. Koenig.
  p. cm.
  Includes bibliographical references and index.
  ISBN 1-932031-55-3 (pbk : alk. paper)
  1. Medicine—Religious aspects. 2. Medical personnel—Religious life. I. Koenig, Harold
George. II. Title.
BL65.M4 C375 2004
261.8'321—dc22
                           2003016620

Printed in the United States of America
04 05 06 07 08 09   10 9 8 7 6 5 4 3 2 1

To J. C. and J. C. C., the two most important men in my life.

To C. M. K. and R. M. K., the two most important women in my life.

Contents

Preface

In today's climate of increasing technological advances, cumbersome insurance procedures, mazes of federal and state regulations, require-ments for additional documentation, rising malpractice rates and esca-lating numbers of legal suits, the looming threat of Medicare and Medicaid collapse, and demands to see more patients, complete more medical tasks, do more with fewer resources, and keep up with the gains in health-related knowledge, we are overwhelmed and exhausted! As hard as we are working, we realize that many who need care are being left behind—and that the delivery of healthcare is becoming increas-ingly difficult. In fact, it is so difficult that some healthcare professionals are asking themselves: Why am I doing this? What is my purpose? Am I making a difference with the patients I serve? Is there a better way? And if there is a better way, what is it?

At the heart of these questions is deep concern. Everyone entering healthcare expects the job to be challenging. How could it not be? Daily we have encounters with those who are wounded and broken by disease—physical, emotional, cognitive, and spiritual disease. These peo-ple look to us for healing, for advice, for comfort and solace. When we find that we are too busy, too tired, and too pulled by what seem to be tangential issues to be fully present to our patients, we experience a sense of "dis-ease." We ask, Where is the joy in serving? How can we recapture the initial dream that motivated us to enter the healthcare professions?

This book examines the *spiritual vision* that initially motivated and continues to nourish many caregivers. We examine this vision through the personal narratives of physicians, nurses, chaplains, healthcare educators, community resource workers, administrators, therapists, psychologists, and social workers. These professionals come from a wide range of religious traditions: Protestant Christianity, Catholic Christianity, Judaism, Islam, Sikhism, Hinduism, Buddhism, and others. The book addresses a number of issues, such as whether the healthcare professional has responded to a felt "call" from God to pursue a particular specialty. We asked participants to reflect on God's continuing influence years after that choice was made. We look at healthcare not as a business concerned with the bottom line but rather as a *ministry* and what that ministry means to patients.

Many may react with discomfort to the idea that healthcare is a ministry, believing that the term *ministry* belongs to the clergy—priests, ministers, chaplains, rabbis—and to members of religious orders. Many would argue that years of professional education and training serve to mold the scientific, objective, and sometimes interpersonal distance that contributes to "good" science.

Yet for many healthcare professionals, there is so much more. Ministry is at the heart of what they do, and at the heart of ministry is service, comfort, relief of pain, healing, and support when healing is not possible. This ministry, supported by prayer, is descriptive of healthcare rooted in spirituality.

We examine the state of the current healthcare system and its impact on the spiritual well-being of those who work in it. We envision an ideal healthcare system that supports and nurtures the spirituality not only of patients and their families but also of the professional caregivers that work to bring about healing, comfort, and solace. We present examples of where elements of the ideal healthcare system already exist.

We provide an overview of the preparation necessary for healthcare professionals to provide spiritual care for patients and families. We take a close look at what spiritual care looks like when we are providing that care for others. We focus on a number of healthcare issues with major spiritual implications, including those with chronic illnesses such as AIDS and dementia; those with psychiatric conditions who may feel abandoned not only by family and society but by God as well; those who are facing death as well as those who are left behind; those with devastating injuries; those facing surgery; and those who live with chronic pain. In each of these healthcare situations there are spiritual threads such as loss and grief, forgiveness, anger, questions of meaning and purpose, and the "Why" questions—Why me? Why now? and Why, God?

Also explored are ways that we as caregivers can maintain our own spiritual health. Activities such as praying alone or with other health professionals, worshiping, taking time to read inspirational literature, going on a retreat, becoming an active member of a faith community, listening to patients in an effort to meet their spiritual needs, and practicing the presence of God while at work are all ways that we can remain spiritually alive and well.

Last, in the appendixes we provide resources for professional caregivers on the beliefs and practices of different religions, assessment tools that can be used in clinical practice, and lists of organizations and other resources that can support health professionals in their roles as spiritual caregivers. Throughout each chapter we include reflective questions and suggestions to assist the healthcare professional in renewing the spiritual focus of practice.

Woven throughout this content are the stories of those who are providing healthcare from a spiritual foundation. We believe in the power of the story—not only the stories of our patients but our own as well. These stories are inspirational and educational and provide a glimpse into the character and motivation of the storyteller. They represent the generous sharing of sixty-five healthcare professionals from a broad array of faith traditions. Regardless of the faith tradition, we heard similar stories of hearing God's call, responding to that call, and carrying forth the message to those who are served. We are grateful to those who generously gave of their time to answer our questions and to share with us.

Our wish is that as you read this book, you will derive certain benefits. First, we hope you will realize that you are not alone. Many struggle with feeling overwhelmed laboring in this chaotic healthcare system, and yet they have been able to overcome discouragement and exhaustion by adopting a spiritual attitude toward their work. There are many who quietly and powerfully provide care based on knowledge of and a relationship with God. They provide loving and compassionate ministrations in spite of the demands of the system in which they function. Second, we hope you will examine your own practice of healthcare and identify ways that your spirituality influences that practice. Third, we ask you to examine ways that you can consciously and systematically influence the healthcare system to return to a vision that embraces and celebrates the spirituality of all.

One consistent theme emerged from all the contributors to this book: that the healthcare system needs to change. The changes that are needed are not cosmetic, nor do they represent minor tweaking of a system that is relatively okay. No, the changes that are imagined are sea changes that relegate technological advances and bureaucratic requirements to a subordinate position, beneath the caring relationship held together with spiritual twine that is at the heart of real healthcare ministry.

You may be thinking that such a change is truly a David-versus-Goliath scenario, that only someone out of touch with reality would even consider such a thing. But there are those who are devoting their professional careers to changing the system in just this way. And there are those such as the professionals whose stories appear in this book who are quietly changing the healthcare system, one day at a time, one patient at a time.

As you begin to read this book and reflect on these stories, consider this story:

ONE AT A TIME

A friend of ours was walking down a deserted Mexican beach at sunset. As he walked along, he began to see another man in the distance. As he grew nearer, he noticed that the local native kept leaning down, picking up something, and throwing it into the water. Time and again he kept hurling things out into the ocean.

As our friend approached even closer, he noticed that the man was picking up starfish that had been washed up on the beach, and one at a time, he was throwing them back into the water.

Our friend was puzzled. He approached the man and said, "Good evening, friend. I was wondering what you are doing."

"I'm throwing these starfish back into the ocean. You see, it's low tide right now and all of these starfish have been washed up onto the shore. If I don't throw them back into the sea, they'll die up here from lack of oxygen."

"I understand," our friend replied, "but there must be thousands of starfish on this beach. You can't possibly get to all of them. There are simply too many. And don't you realize this is probably happening on hundreds of beaches all up and down this coast? Can't you see that you can't possibly make a difference?"

The local native smiled, bent down, and picked up yet another starfish, and as he threw it back into the sea, he replied, "Made a difference to that one!"

—Author Unknown

Verna Benner Carson, Ph.D., APRN/PMH
Harold G. Koenig, M.D.

Acknowledgments

Very few accomplishments are completed without help from others, and this book is no exception. The first group that deserves our thanks is the healthcare professionals who shared their stories with us. Without their generous contributions there would be no book. We asked them a lot of questions; we asked to hear long, in-depth stories; we asked very busy people to share their time with us. Without exception, we got what we asked for. We believe it is important to thank them each by name, and so we thank each of them here and include a list of their names in the list of contributors.

Thanks to Martha Loveland, a nurse and healthcare administrator who offered the perspective of "management" on what is needed to make the work environment more spiritual. Thank you to Drs. Julie Steiner, Herman Brecher, Bernita Taylor, and Franz Sewchand from Seton Medical Group in Catonsville, Maryland. Their stories of call and care are peppered throughout the book. Deep appreciation to Dr. Christina Puchalski for sharing with us her story of call and how she is turning her commitment to spiritual care into a reality at George Washington University. Dr. Gunnar E. Christiansen, a retired ophthalmologist who presently volunteers his time at the National Alliance for the Mentally Ill, shared deeply touching reflections from his career. To the psychiatric nurses, Nancy Shoemaker, Evelyn Yapp, Cynthia Poort, and Vicki Germer, who work with the "sickest of the sick and poorest of the poor" and do so with love and compassion, never forgetting the importance of their patients' spiritual needs—thank you. Thanks to Joyce Kinstlinger, a community resource counselor, who shared her calling to work with the most unfortunate in society. To Miriam Jacik, retired oncology nurse who continues to give to the bereaved, your insights were priceless. Thanks to Sandra Brown, family nurse practitioner, who strives to weave her spirituality into every interaction. To Shirley Herron, spiritual director and consultant regarding palliative care, your moving impressions of the icebergs off the coast of Newfoundland remind us that we can encounter God in the beauty of his creations.

Thanks to Dr. Sagrid Eleanor Edman, retired nursing dean of Bethel College, who always wanted to be a nurse and even asked Santa to bring her mother white nylons so her mom could look like a nurse! Dr. Edman has channeled her calling into the support of parish nursing. Our thanks go out to Dr. Patricia Camp, a retired nursing faculty member, who also continues to respond to God's call through her work in parish nursing. Recognition goes to another retired nursing dean, Dr. Sandra Jamison, who went into nursing because she greatly admired the work of her physician father. Dr. Jamison continues her commitment to nursing through the graduate ministry of Nurses' Christian Fellowship. Dr. Karen Soeken, a non-nurse faculty member, gave her perspective on what makes a work environment a spiritual place; she shared how the call of God for her to teach has been a constant throughout her career. Harriet Coeling, a nursing faculty member, told us how the current healthcare environment makes her more aware of her need to maintain a relationship with God and to draw upon God for strength and guidance. Genie Ford, also involved in nursing education, did not want to be a nurse, but God not only called her, he pushed her into nursing!

Thank you to Chaplain Jeffrey Flowers, whose story of Cassie, the baby who lived only one hour and twelve minutes, reminded us that it is not the length of a life nor the accomplishments of that life that make it valuable, but rather it is the presence of God in that life. To Reverend Rodger Murchison, whose work with the bereaved is a powerful spiritual intervention—we thank you for sharing. To Chaplain Robb Small, thank you for reminding us that to stay spiritually healthy we need to pray and play often! To Dr. Don Berry, dear friend, minister, and founder and president of the Institute for Religion and Health, thank you for your beautiful words regarding your own calling to serve God.

Charity Johansson, our only physical therapy participant, moved us greatly with her account of her "evolving" call, her struggles to meet the needs of the institution and at the same time be a spiritual presence to her patients, and her great desire that the workplace support openly sanctioned time for renewal of body, soul, and spirit. And, Jay Brashear, our only occupational therapist, challenges us all to make sure we are truly caring for the patient and not the chart. Jay's description of how he approaches every patient's bath as if he were assisting the Lord himself is an image that can help us all when we are feeling too tired to give.

Sister Karen Pozniak gave us an excellent example of how God may change our call over time as she described the evolution of her call from religious life, to working with the sick and dying, to becoming a chaplain who teaches volunteers to work with the sick and dying. Nurse Elizabeth Page also experienced a changing call, beginning her nursing ministry in the hospital, then moving to a nursing home ministry and currently working with handicapped children and their families.

Physician Daniel Ober shared his experiences working as a hospice medical director and told us how he ministers to suffering people out of his own spiritual resources. Retired pediatric hematologist and oncologist Alton Lightsey related how he often served as a mediator between the child who was his patient and the child's parent to help resolve spiritual end-of-life issues.

Dr. Michael Parker, who focuses his social work and psychology background on the care of the elderly, gives us a wonderful example as he strives to affirm the faith of the elderly and encourages them to continue to serve communities and families. Dr. Othelia Lee, another social worker, shares her efforts to integrate spirituality into her teaching as well as her interactions with peers. We are thankful for those who reach out to others.

Thanks to Eileen Altenhofer, Carol Story, Carole Kornelis, Catherine Lick, Kay Hurd, and Kelly Preston, each involved in some aspect of parish nursing and each with powerful stories of how they minister to others. Thanks to nurses Beatrice Rosen, Marilyn Bulloch, Ada Scharf, Charmin Koenig, Nancy Hines, and Diane Molitor—each contributed memorable examples of their own spiritual ministry to patients.

Diane's affirmation, "God is the real deal, we should be too," is a reminder to us of the importance of authenticity in all relationships. Thanks to Dee Brooks, Carole Richards, and Dianne Smith, all of whom specialize in pediatric nursing, for reminding us that sick children and their families are in need of our ministry.

Physician Jack Hasson, as well as nurses Susan Feldman and Margie Schmier, explained how they approach spirituality from a Jewish perspective. We were moved by each of their stories. Surgeon Tom Grace's willingness to pray with his patients reminds us how important prayer is for surgical patients.

We are grateful to the physicians and psychologists who provided us with Islamic, Buddhist, Hindu, and Sikh perspectives on spirituality. It is clear from their stories that God calls each of us—we need only listen. Physicians Tarif Bakdash, Jirpesh Patel, Shahid Athar, and Hasan Shanawani, we thank you for the Islamic view. Thanks also to Reverend Kong Chhean, a psychologist and Buddhist monk, who has dedicated his life to assisting Cambodians in their healing from traumatic memories. Dr. Shyam Bhat, we thank you as well for providing us a Hindu perspective on receiving a calling. We appreciate the story of Dr. T. D. Singh, who heard God's voice in the midst of grieving his mother's unexpected death. Thank you, Dr. Dharma Singh Khalsa, for sharing your experience of receiving more than one call.

Nurses Amy Pollman, Florie Miranda, Brenda Thornton, and Karen McCauley provided us with a homecare perspective. Amy's recollection of singing "Friends in High Places" for a patient who had just lost her husband will stay with us a long time. Karen's story of how a dying patient ministered to her reminds us that we receive as much from patients as we give. Florie's narrative of her ministry to a young man dying from AIDS reminds us of the importance of leaving no one out of our ministry. Brenda's story of her faithfulness as she worked with angry Floyd reminds us that absolutely no one is immune from the transforming power of love.

We are thankful for all the patients and families whose stories we also heard throughout the text. It is clear again that they minister to us as we to them. Thanks to Kathy Guiffrida, who transcribed the taped interviews—a tedious but necessary task. Thanks to John Carson, who helped find appropriate opening quotations for each of the chapters. Thanks to Laura Barrett of Templeton Foundation Press for her patience in waiting for the final manuscript.

Throughout the text we talk about the power of prayer, and the completion of this book is a tribute to that power. We had people praying for us all over the country. That prayer provided inspiration and support when the words just didn't want to come. We are so thankful to have a network of dependable "pray-ers."

We want to end these acknowledgments with the refrain of a hymn entitled "We Are Called." The words speak to the responsiveness of each of the professionals represented in this text.

> We are called to act with justice
> We are called to love tenderly
> We are called to serve one another
> To walk humbly with God.[1]

Spiritual Caregiving

[1]

Spiritual Caregiving
Healthcare as a Ministry

A life devoted to things is a dead life, a stump;
a God-shaped life is a flourishing tree.
                                        —*The Message*

HEALTHCARE AS MINISTRY

This chapter presents stories told by doctors, nurses, chaplains, physical therapists, and other health professionals, discussing the concept of ministry as it pertains to healthcare, exploring the sense of call that led them into their chosen fields, examining how they define spirituality and religion, and describing how their spirituality and/or religious beliefs influence their daily work.

Many may react with discomfort to the idea that healthcare is a ministry, believing that the term "ministry" belongs to the clergy—priests, ministers, chaplains, rabbis—and to members of religious orders. Many would argue that years of professional education and training serve to mold the scientific, objective, and sometimes interpersonal distance that contributes to "good" science.

Yet for many healthcare professionals, there is so much more.

Ministry is at the heart of what they do, and at the heart of ministry is service, comfort, relief of pain, healing, and support when healing is not possible. This ministry, supported by prayer, is descriptive of healthcare rooted in spirituality.

Oncology nurse Miriam Jacik believes that the focus of a profession and a ministry are slightly different, and that with the profession comes a "setting apart" of the helper from the person being helped. Catholic theologian Henri Nouwen, in a similar vein, observes that with increasing professionalization comes a widening space between the professional and the patient. This widening space tends to produce in the patient feelings of intimidation, fear, and apprehension toward the more powerful professional.[1] Patients may believe that the education and training of the professional have endowed him or her with mysterious power. Patients view healthcare providers with a mixture of fear and awe, accepting that the professional uses a language that cannot be understood, does things that cannot be questioned, and often makes decisions about patients' lives with no explanations.[2] The poor, who already bear a disproportionate amount of suffering, are especially subject to these emotions. Many leave places of supposed healing feeling physically better but hurt by the interpersonal treatment they received at the hands of a healthcare provider.

This situation is not totally the fault of the healthcare professional, who is often the first to recognize the challenge of remaining interpersonally open to patients. The healer is under increased demands to do more, see more patients, complete more paperwork, deal with more bureaucratic requirements for payment, be aware of changing healthcare regulations, and remain current on advances in healthcare. The challenge to healthcare providers committed to ministry is great and requires constant striving to develop a personal spirituality that energizes them with purpose and meaning, enables them to find the time to ease the interpersonal pain experienced by so many of their patients, and protects them from excessively absorbing and becoming immobilized by that pain.[3]

CHARACTERISTICS OF A MINISTERING PERSON

Carol Story, a parish nurse, shares an experience of ministry:

On one occasion I was talking to a patient dying with cancer. This man had earned his Ph.D. and had dedicated his life to teaching. He was questioning the value of his life—had he made a difference? What did his life mean? We spoke for a long time about his life. He shared a painful experience that occurred when he was fifteen years old. A pastor had embarrassed him in front of the congregation by berating him, predicting that he would never be anything or anybody of significance. He reflected that he had taught a few students who moved on to be leaders in sports and education.

As I listened to all he shared, I synthesized what I was hearing. "What I am hearing you say is that you always felt unworthy of any praise because of what one man said to you as a young man." He looked at me and said, "Yes, you have put into words something that I have struggled with for years—but it is true. I have always wondered if I measured up and felt unworthy. Thank you." Then I simply said, "May I give you a message from God?" He replied, "Yes." I said, "God loves you, and I believe he is going to say, 'Well done, thou good and faithful servant!'" He grabbed my hand and said with tears, "Thank you," and then asked me to pray with him.

Carol Story provided good nursing and good ministry.

Thankfully, there are many who practice every day, in hospitals, clinics, offices, homes, nursing homes, and professional schools, motivated by a powerful call—a sense of rightness about what they do. Each of these professionals draws from a deep personal spiritual well that keeps them nourished and allows them to minister to patients, families, co-workers, and even institutions.

In her examination of medicine as a ministry, Margaret E. Mohrmann, a physician, believes that the care of suffering persons requires that caregivers, drawn from within and beyond the ranks of the medical profession, acknowledge and honor the life stories of those to whom we provide care.[4] Mohrmann emphasizes that God loves us as unique persons, each precious in his eyes. We have different needs, different problems, and different stories, so that honoring each of our stories requires

At the heart of being a ministering person is seeking to hear and understand the story of the suffering person standing before us and to encourage hope in that person in developing the next chapter of the story.

❧

A ministering person enters into a relationship with another and shares that individual's pain, listens even when it causes some inconvenience, says little or nothing, and at other times raises questions for reflection.

a personal approach and a relationship that recognizes and responds to our uniqueness. At the heart of being a ministering person is seeking to hear and understand the story of the suffering person standing before us and to encourage hope in that person in developing the next chapter of the story.

Let's examine the specific characteristics of ministering healthcare professionals who seek to hear and respond to the stories of patients.[5]

The first characteristic is the ability to enter into a relationship with another and share that individual's pain, to listen even when it causes some inconvenience, to say little or nothing and at other times to raise questions for reflection. Physician Jack Hasson states, "My own spirituality makes me more sensitive to others. When I recognize that a patient or family has a desire to express their spiritual needs, I try to allow this expression without applying my own belief system. They know best what works for their spirituality, and I allow myself to be a conduit for their feelings and pain. I will then amplify and confirm their belief if possible." This is a good example of allowing space for the other's beliefs and pain. It is in this space that the patient and healthcare provider can reach out to each other and "connect as fellow travelers sharing the same broken human condition."[6]

The second characteristic of ministering persons is that they take the role of companion to another's journey rather than problem solver or rescuer. This involves serious reflection about the concerns of the patient, being present when needs arise, and sensing that we share a sense of helplessness and brokenness with the one we are helping. Miriam Jacik recounts:

As an oncology nurse I had frequent occasion to see and experience patients and their family members grappling with the meaning of illness, suffering, and death.

Helping them ask their own questions and arrive at their own answers in time was a spiritual service that I could offer. Seeing them turn from anger at a God who would let terrible things happen to good people, to seeking strength and comfort needed from that same God, always strengthened the faith of all of us. Helping family members let go and release their loved ones to the process of death and into the arms of the God of their beliefs was a spiritual service that my personal beliefs and values allowed me to provide.

A ministering person takes the role of companion to another's journey rather than being a problem solver or rescuer.

The third characteristic of a ministering person is the ability to love the unlovable, the ungrateful, the uncooperative, the aggressive, and the unreachable. Charmin Koenig tells a story of a challenging patient for whom she provided care.

A ministering person loves the unlovable, the ungrateful, the uncooperative, the aggressive, and the unreachable.

There was one patient, a woman who suffered greatly from migraines. I had such compassion for her—I understand what it is like to suffer from migraines. The rest of the staff were angry with this patient because they believed that she abused the system—she came in so often for pain medication. I saw something different. I wanted to work with her, and of course no one argued with me about this. They were glad that they didn't have to care for her. She was a very angry woman, angry at life, but most of all angry at God. Even though we did not share the same beliefs, I had opportunities to pray with her. I prayed for her healing, but more specifically I prayed for "heart healing." When she came in for care, she always asked that I be her nurse. Over time there was a dramatic change in her attitude—she seemed to soften, to harbor less anger.

The fourth ministering characteristic is that we accept our own brokenness, humanness, and fragility so as to enter into relationship with those who are burdened by the difficulties of life. This allows the freedom to cry with a person in sorrow, to rejoice with one who meets success, to share anger in the face of injustices, and to accept the doubts and confusion caused by the events of life.

Kelly Preston shares a story from early in her nursing career.

A ministering person accepts her own brokenness, humanness, and fragility so as to enter into relationships with those who are burdened by the difficulties of life.

I was working in oncology. One night a man was admitted with a serious heart condition but also terminal leukemia. Within twelve hours of being admitted, he was dead. We were unsure of his code status, and when he experienced a cardiac arrest, we initiated a code on him. We shouldn't have. I felt awful about the whole situation, that he died so quickly, that we put him through the trauma of the code. I just felt the pain of it. When I saw his wife and daughter, they embraced me, and we cried and prayed together. They told me that it meant so much to them that I was present to them and not afraid to share my emotions.

The fifth ministering characteristic is to be a facilitator of change in others but not assume responsibility for that change. Let's listen to Chaplain Robb Small's story.

I ministered to a middle-aged woman who suffered from mental health issues, including depression and anxiety. When I first met her, she talked constantly, ending every sentence with a catch phrase, "But God will never put more on a person that that person can bear, don't you agree?" For some reason, I chose not to verbally answer her and instead sat and listened attentively for a long time with only occasional head nods or other gestures. After about an hour of this, the patient stopped and asked me if this was the way I ministered, just sitting and saying nothing. I replied that I felt that she needed to talk more than listen to me. At first she became angry and stated that I was supposed to be the helper and that I was called to fix her problems. Over time she became angrier that I would not respond with "God talk."

After a few visits, she asked me one day what gave me the ability to resist telling her what to do or believe. It was easy at this point to explain that in my spiritual experience, her greatest need was to discover the answers from within herself, and my job was to facilitate that process with whatever resources I could bring to the relationship without giving advice. The most important role I could offer was to listen attentively, be present, unconditionally accept her condition, and share God's love and grace.

The sixth ministering characteristic is to allow others to make decisions and support them through that process. Martha Loveland shares a story about a hospice patient who preferred not to have further medical treatment or heroic care.

A ministering person facilitates change in others but does not assume responsibility for that change.

The patient's spiritual beliefs allowed him to be accepting and peaceful about his impending death. He did ask to have his pain reduced as much as possible. However, his son insisted that he participate in a research protocol. The son did not state his motives for this position, and his insistence was distressing to his father. Because of my spiritually based valuing of both of them, I was able to bridge the gap between them. I assured the patient that what he wanted could be arranged and would be the basis of the plan of care. I assured the son that his father loved him and the family, was not desirous of dying, but didn't want to be an unnecessary burden. I also stressed that his father had the right to choose the manageable conditions surrounding his impending death. I explained to the son that this right was extended to everyone and protected by federal law, the Patient Self-Determination Act. I taught the son ways he could support his father and enjoy the remaining time as much as possible.

The seventh ministering characteristic is to accept that solutions to problems are best arrived at by the person being served. Cynthia Ann Poort describes an experience of working with a patient with AIDS and how, through her presence and nonjudgmental listening, he was able to resolve painful personal memories and restore broken relationships.

A ministering person allows others to make decisions and supports them through the decision-making process.

When I was a staff nurse, I cared for an AIDS patient who was slowly dying. He received a two-hour intravenous infusion daily. My job was to start the infusion, remain in the home, draw blood work, and leave after discontinuing the infusion. I was in his home for two hours daily for about two months. We spoke of many different topics as we waited for the IV to infuse. He expressed a great deal of anger toward his father, who had been a church deacon. The patient believed his father was a

A ministering person accepts that solutions to problems are best arrived at by the person being served.

ॐ

A ministering person is able to recognize that one cannot put an end to the psychological pain and suffering of others, but can be a witness to it and give voice to that suffering.

hypocrite because he had an affair with another woman while his mother was dying. The patient stated that he hated "Christians" for this reason. He told me that his father had married the woman with whom he had the affair, and to show his anger toward his father, the patient showed up in "full drag" at the conservative church wedding.

My patient was alienated from all his family members except for a grandmother who occasionally called on the phone. His former significant other had died of AIDS about one year earlier. I was able to listen to my patient and help him deal with his anger, grief, and alienation from his spiritual upbringing and his family. He came to realize that spirituality and the form of religious beliefs that one espouses may not be the same thing. He reconnected with his grandmother, who had great faith, and was able to come to terms with his anger toward his father. He really had not wanted to deny his faith, but had done so out of his anger toward his father. He was able to forgive his father even though his father was now dead and was able to prepare for death and feel some peace in his life.

The eighth ministering characteristic is the ability to recognize that one cannot put an end to others' psychological pain and suffering, but can be a witness to it and give voice to that suffering. Dr. Gunnar Christiansen shares his experiences as a volunteer working with the mentally ill: "It is not uncommon to have questions from those with a serious mental illness, such as, 'God, why me?' and 'What did I do to deserve this?' Although I do not feel that we have answers to these questions, I feel that it is helpful to discuss the questions. In my experience, I believe I have been more helpful in these discussions with those individuals who share my faith."

The ninth characteristic of a ministering person is the ability to accept others the way they are and make no attempt to fashion them into different people.

Carol Story shares her experience working with an elderly gentleman who expressed views very different from her own beliefs.

On one occasion, I was talking to a ninety-year-old man who told me that his mother had been Catholic. He asked me if I was Catholic or a nun. When I said no, he launched into his story. He was cognitively alert, very expressive and direct as he told his story. "When I was a little boy of ten, someone at my school made me bow down on my knees, and I had to kiss his ring. I vowed that I was never going to bow down to another man. So I refused to go to that school anymore. But I was faithful to my mother. I took her to church up until she died." He paused and said, "Her face glowed when leaving church." I asked him, "Where did that glow come from?" He said, "You know where it came from."

He continued with his story as tears began to roll down his cheeks. He told me how he had raised his children around the table on the Bible. "You know there are some parts of that Bible that aren't true. For instance, God made man in his own image. Well, you know that isn't true. God is spirit and we aren't." He then changed the topic to tell me that he learned to meditate from his daughter. I asked him, "Would you tell me how you meditate?" He explained this to me, and then we sat in silence.

I began to pray that the Lord would give me something to say, and suddenly I said, "Can we talk about your mom for a minute?" He said yes. Then I gently touched his chest and asked, "What were you feeling in here when those tears came down your cheeks?" He looked at me, and, with tears again, said, "Broken." And I asked, "What would it take to fix it?" Brushing the tears away, he looked at me, shook his finger in my face, and said, "You!" I said, "Me?" He said, "Yes! You sitting here listening to me, believing that I am not just an old man who doesn't have a brain and that I can't think for myself. No one has to tell me what I believe, because I know what I believe."

We both sat there for a minute, and then I thanked him for sharing with me. He asked me to pray for his wife, and during the prayer I asked God to bless this gentleman for sharing his faith with me.

> A ministering person is able to accept others the way they are and make no attempt to fashion them into different people.

The tenth and last ministering characteristic is the ability to encourage others to delineate their own values, goals, and personal views. Martha Loveland, a nurse and healthcare administrator, exemplifies this

A ministering person is able to encourage others to delineate their own values, goals, and personal views. ministering characteristic in her approach to employees: "It is critical to understand that humans have God-given choice. In balancing the needs of the employer with employee choice, the employer-employee relationship is strengthened by clear understanding of job expectations/duties and policies/procedures, especially at the time of hire. For example, if abortions are performed in a facility, Catholic staff need full information about this as well as other provided services that might conflict with their belief system."

REFLECTIONS

- How would you describe your ability to encourage and honor the stories of suffering persons?
- What are your own experiences of having your personal story encouraged and honored? What value did these experiences have for you?
- Which of the ten characteristics of a ministering person do you most embody? Which characteristics are the most troublesome for you to practice?
- Can you think of specific ways that you can make your healthcare practice more of a healing ministry?

CHOOSING A PROFESSION: RESPONDING TO A CALL

Roslyn Karaban contends that at the essence of a call to ministry is the story of an encounter between an individual and God.[7] When we asked health professionals, "Did you experience a call to your profession?" the responses were quite varied. Sometimes they found it difficult to discern the voice of God amid the clamor and noise of daily life. Unlike the demands of family and employers, whose call to us is demanding, the call of God is loving and gentle, and can be ignored and pushed aside. We are each called to love and honor God in the unique roles that we fulfill, in chosen vocations and avocations, in volunteer activity, in quiet time, and most of all in relationships.[8]

Many of those that we queried were emphatic in their sense of call. Some were not aware of having that experience at all. Others looked back after the choice of profession was made and recognized God's voice calling them. Among those who felt called, the sense of that call varied. To some of them God's summons was heard as a general call to a life of service. To others, God's summons was a specific call to their chosen profession. Let's look at how respondents explained how and why they entered their particular profession.

Dr. Bernita Taylor describes her choice of medicine as a career: "I always wanted to be of service, and I found medicine fascinating. I guess I wanted to be like Marcus Welby. He was a super doc. As I look back, I didn't recognize a call to be a doctor, but I do know that God got me through medical school and residency. I didn't do it alone."

> Everyone is called to love and honor God in the unique roles that he or she fulfills, in chosen vocations and avocations, in volunteer activity, in quiet time, and most of all in relationships. At the heart of a call to minister is a personal encounter between an individual and God, leading to an unfolding story of service.

Dianne Smith grew up in a family with many physicians who served as role models, providing Dianne with a sense of comfort and belonging in the hospital setting:

I began volunteering in my great-uncle's hospital (he helped start it) as a teenager. I was very comfortable around sick people, and I enjoyed helping them. I also enjoyed science and math and began college as a pre-med student. I soon realized that I didn't want to go to school for as long as it would take to be a doctor, and I also wanted a closer tie with patients. I thought nursing would give me this. I didn't feel called when I chose nursing, but shortly after entering nursing, I felt that this was what God wanted for me.

The call has grown stronger over the years. I have done inpatient pediatric nursing for twenty-one years and have dealt with some very challenging situations. I'm often the one who is asked to take the difficult assignment, and I feel very comfortable with this. Whenever another job opportunity has come along, whether it is an "easier" aspect of nursing or something outside of nursing, I have felt a strong message from God to continue with what I am doing.

Psychologist Kong Chhean shares his story:

I was born and raised in a Buddhist family in Cambodia. I was committed to a Buddhist temple when I was a child. In 1968 I finished my studies at the Buddhist University in Phnom Penh, Cambodia. I then left Cambodia to study Buddhism and psychology in India, where I became a Theravada Buddhist monk. In 1989, when I moved to the Long Beach area in California in the United States, the first thing I did was to build a Buddhist temple. I am the spiritual leader of the Cambodian Buddhists in Long Beach. After building the temple, I returned to school to obtain an M.A. in counseling psychology from Pepperdine University in 1986 and a Ph.D. in clinical psychology from American Commonwealth University in 1989.

I felt a spiritual calling to help my people in the combined roles of Buddhist monk and psychologist. Many Cambodians desire to hold onto their Buddhist way of life, and they need assistance in dealing with the conflict they face in their new society as they attempt to preserve the past and adapt to the present. For many Cambodians who have come to the United States after surviving the traumatic war in Cambodia from 1975 to 1979, Buddhist monks play an important role in psychotherapy, in Eastern and Western family therapy, and in restoring the Cambodians to their lost health.

"Yes, I felt called," Charity Johansson recalls.

However, it took a while to discern the specifics of the calling. There were several areas of interest for me, but I had to choose one that I felt morally good exchanging money for. I examined my gifts from different perspectives, then chose the one that I felt most "led" in. Once I was at Stamford Physical Therapy School, I had one of those rare moments in which I knew that I was where I was supposed to be.

Although the call has evolved over the years, it has never lost its essence. Early in my career, geriatrics and education held special interest for me, but I thought I would be content forever as a staff physical therapist. But it's as if following a call requires a certain amount of venturing forth into the unknown. To the degree that pursuing the call is an act of faith, steps forward must often be made in the presence of and in spite of some fog! My practice has grown from nearly 100 percent hands-on traditional technique in an institutional setting to much more of a "guide" role. I'm an educator now, teaching physical therapy, doing some hands-on practice, but specializing in less traditional techniques and finding a voice for my own unique contributions to my profession.

After entering medical school, Dr. Shahid Athar recognized God's call on his life.

Although I was born into a Muslim family and knew Islamic rituals, I did not discover God until I started to reflect upon His creation, especially the human body. At age nineteen, as I dissected cadavers in medical school, looking at the arrangements and purpose of bone, nerves, vessels, organs, and their interconnection and function, it began to impress me that this machine could not have created itself. I was reading the human body as a book, trying to locate the author. I appreciated the masterpiece painting and asked: Where is the artist? . . . Once I found God by reason, I wanted to know more about Him and asked myself: What does God want me to do? What aspects of my life does He influence?[9]

Evelyn Yapp, a psychiatric nurse, notes, "There were many factors that influenced my choice of nursing. Initially, to be honest, I did not realize the calling. On very deep reflection I realize that God gently and softly led me to fulfill my vision of following in the footsteps of the Lord through servitude, devotion, and sacrifices. As I dealt with the impact of many losses in my own life, it dawned on me that God was calling me to witness what it is to be in deepest communion with him through nursing."

Child psychiatrist Jirpesh Patel adds, "I didn't receive a 'call from God' per se, but when I was doing my psychiatry residency, I became fascinated with child psychiatry. I wanted to help children who were struggling emotionally in the current challenging environment. My Hindu priest helped me consolidate my instinct to make this decision. Now I am happy to be serving children."

Although Dee Brooks knew she wanted to be a nurse from a very early age, she did not recognize the voice of God calling her.

I loved science and wanted to know what made the human body tick. As I have matured, I have come to know and appreciate my spiritual nature and to explore my walk with the Lord. I now realize that what I received was a calling, and a very special one. I work with sick children and feel distinctly honored that God entrusted this work to me for the last thirty-one years. I am grateful every day for my nursing career. The wondrous souls that have passed my way are priceless treasures in the forms of my patients and their families, as well as friends and co-workers in the medical field. Every day I go to work, I see God's face and feel God's love surrounding me.

Dr. T. D. Singh, a chemist who is also involved in counseling, shares this experience.

In April 1979, by the mercy of the Supreme Lord, I received an inner call while I was working on my Ph.D. in chemistry at the University of California at Irvine. One day I received an unexpected telegram from my home in India stating that my mother had passed away. This came as a complete shock to me, for I had no prior information that she was even ill. This event acted as a catalyst for this experience of the "call": This material world is filled with uncertainties and unpredictable sufferings, and I should search for a lasting spiritual and divine meaning of life and help others do the same. This is enunciated in the Vedic literatures of India. Over the years my "call" has intensified my commitment to pursue a career of helping others through a holistic approach to life—that is, through scientific, spiritual, and religious experience.

Nancy Shoemaker reflects, "I always wanted to become a nurse. Nurses who cared for me as a child influenced me, as well as my mother, who told me when I graduated that she herself had always wanted to be a nurse. I do feel that nursing is a calling, and I view the care of my patients as a sacred trust. I have now practiced psychiatric nursing for more than thirty years, and I have never regretted my decision about my career. I still strive for excellence today, just as I did when I first graduated."

Psychiatrist Shyam Bhat explains his sense of calling:

As a Hindu, I was always exposed to the belief that suffering, and by extension mental and physical illness, is predestined by karmic fate—something irrevocable and therefore to be endured. My interest in psychiatry and medicine was not inspired by a sudden "calling" from God; it was partly intellectual, and partly as a reaction to the prevalent stigma against mental illness that exists in India, and perhaps in most other parts of the world.

However, over the years, I have had a growing awareness that there has to be a sense to all that we do, a purpose, and in contemplating those issues, I have become more aware about how my spirituality affects my experience and practice of my profession. So, I experienced no epiphany, no sudden realization that this was what I was created to do. Instead, I have experienced a gradual (and still evolving) belief that in some spiritual way, my task is to do what I do to the best of my ability, with little thought about external reactions (or lack of them).

Harriet Coeling remembers,

I became a nurse because as a high school student I enjoyed volunteering in a hospital and helping people feel better. I also was impressed with the complexity of coordinating all the efforts of all the employees in a hospital and wanted to help "schedule" things so that the work flowed smoothly. I felt called to nursing in the sense that God certainly approved of my going into nursing and could use me in nursing, but I did not feel that the call was exclusively to nursing but rather to several other professions, such as becoming a teacher or a librarian.

Over the years, my sense of calling has definitely become stronger and more focused as I see how God has given me unique abilities that I can use for him. God has been preparing me throughout my life for the opportunities he is now giving me in nursing. Today I can see more clearly how he has nurtured my desire to help others and my leadership skills to be used in nursing "at such a time as this." What a joy to see how God has been at work throughout my career, even when I was unaware of his actions!

Internist Julie Steiner recalls how "even as a child, I wanted to be in the medical field. I like being able to help people in need and felt that I could handle the enormous responsibility that came with caring for the sick. I didn't feel called in a religious sense but more in a humanistic sense."

Dr. Karen Soeken recognized that God had given her the gift of teaching. Although she never sought out teaching opportunities in the health professions, when opportunity knocked at her door and "it felt right," she flung open the door and embraced the opportunity! Dr. Soeken explains that the sense of rightness combined with the opportunity is what she considers a call. Over the years the idea that God has called her to teach has never changed.

Internist Christina Puchalski describes her calling:

The whole concept of being of service to others has always been important to me, so when it came time for me to think about what I would do with my life, the idea of becoming a doctor seemed a natural choice. I was always interested in medicine, and I believe it is a tremendous privilege to help people in that way. I am sure that is where my sense of calling comes from. In fact, when I was in college, I had considered becoming a nun, and I remember sitting down with a priest and telling him, "I definitely want to become a physician, but I also want to become a nun." He helped me discern the difference in calling. But I very much, even then, saw medicine as a calling as opposed to just work, and I take the calling of the profession very seriously. I think that I was greatly influenced by values passed onto me from my parents. My family were all really service-oriented people. That value, I think, has been the strongest influence on my decision to be a physician.

CALL TO CHAPLAINCY

Since both Chaplain Jeffrey Flowers's parents were nurses, he was intimately acquainted with the healing professions.

My faith became very important to me as a child, and I felt a strong "calling" to become a vocational minister. It was a natural fit that I would do ministry in a healthcare setting. However, the reasons that I continue to do ministry are not the same ones that led me to it initially. I now believe that my call is to guide people toward wholeness and to build relationships that assist in times of crisis as well as times of prosperity. Initially I felt a strong need to protect the dogma and defend the faith. I see this ministry now as much more of a journey, not a destination.

Chaplain Robb Small describes a lack of direction when he entered the seminary. He accepted a job in a local hospital working in security and knew that the healthcare environment was where he wanted to be.

Soon after taking this job, I discovered my niche and sought special training to remain in the medical field. As a hospital chaplain, I feel a special call to understand the various needs of the sick and also the staff that serve the sick. I feel a call to deal with death and dying, and I am very comfortable in this setting. Although I never felt a "burning bush" type of call, I have always found doors opened that enabled me to serve in the capacity of a chaplain. I will admit that as I look back, I cannot completely claim full responsibility for the grace that enabled me to arrive at this point in my professional development. There has to have been some divine intervention.

Dr. Don Berry is emphatic about his experience:

Yes, I sensed a call to give myself to Christ's ministry in the service to others by using gifts, skills, and longings to fulfill his good purposes. The "call" was always understood as from God and for God, to be used in ministry with and for others. Throughout the years since I was sixteen, the unifying center, the underpinnings of the call have been unwavering. However, the expressions of the call— place, varying kinds of ministry, different arenas of faith and practice—are ever changing: pastor, professor, administrator, writer. But the primary call has always been as a servant of Christ for others.

RESPONDING TO A CHANGING CALL

Sometimes the call changes over time. Sister Karen Pozniak explains:

My first call was to my religious life. Later I got involved with the Charismatic Renewal and working with parents of the children I was teaching. I saw the need to deepen my own faith and ability to share that faith with others. I went on for a master's degree in spirituality. While I was completing my studies, I worked at our infirmary, where I was encouraged by my order to minister to sisters who were sick and dying. After this, I went to a parish with a hospital, and I provided the training for the volunteers who visited the patients at the hospital. Following this experience, I really felt called to become a chaplain. I went to school for clinical pastoral education and took a job as a chaplain. At first I thought I was to provide direct patient care, but as it has turned out, I am using my teaching skills to empower volunteers who visit patients. I am expanding my ministry and helping others to grow spiritually.

Anesthesiologist Dharma Singh Khalsa, speaking from the perspective of a Sikh, shares his changing call:

I have received more than one call. I always had it in my mind to be a physician. I also loved music and played the French horn throughout college. Then one day I had a calling in the sense of awakening one morning realizing that I needed to become a doctor. I stopped playing the horn the next day. After specializing in anesthesiology, I moved to New Mexico, where I met the man I consider to be my spiritual teacher, Yogi Bhajan. When I met him I realized that I no longer had to use powerful drugs to put people to sleep, but rather I could use alternatives such as yoga, meditation, and so on to help them wake up and truly heal. By far my most powerful calling, however, came to me in a dream. I had a visit from God, who told me to write a very particular book and to call it Life without Death: A Doctor's Prescription for Heaven on Earth. *I am working on it now. I am dedicated to helping people bring more spirit into their lives, and to helping doctors become what I call an enlightened healer.*

Miriam Jacik provides another story of a changing call.

My professional life began within the teaching profession. Teaching was the primary ministry of the religious community to which I belonged. Nursing followed teaching, and grew out of a desire to be of "more service" to the handicapped children I was serving at a rehabilitation center in São Paulo, Brazil. Education and training in nursing enabled me to minister to the handicapped and the ill both in the United States and in Brazil, where I spent eleven and a half years. Over time, pastoral counseling became linked to my health ministry. As an oncology nurse, I taught, provided nursing care, and counseled patients dealing with a fatal illness and facing death.

I have felt called to each of the professions I have pursued. These professions developed and became a part of my life as needs and opportunities manifested themselves. Currently, I minister utilizing all the professional training that I possess. As the director of a grief support group that is part of the parish nursing program within my church, I am able to teach and counsel the bereaved.

REFLECTIONS

❧ Did you receive a call to your profession?

❧ How was that call experienced?

❧ Has the nature of that call changed throughout your professional career?

❧ In what ways are you living out the call that you experienced?

RELIGIOUS FAITH AND SPIRITUALITY

More than sixty healthcare professionals shared their stories with us. They represent a broad variety of healthcare specialties, as well as a wide range of faith traditions. We queried the respondents regarding their own faith traditions and how they defined religion and spirituality. Appendix D provides an analysis of professional affiliations and faith traditions.

In response to the question, "How do you define *religion* and *spirituality*?" many of the respondents defined the terms in a similar fashion while drawing comparable distinctions between religion and spirituality, viewing spirituality as the heartfelt experience of God and religion as the attempt to codify and capture that experience.

This distinction is evident in Chaplain Robb Small's definitions:

Spirituality deals with how we are connected in relationship with God. Spirituality has to do with meaning and purpose, and how these factor into being a "holistic" person. If we balance the physical, emotional, and spiritual components, then we tend to enjoy health. In my opinion, spirituality is much like the root word spirit. It is within us, around us, about us—every aspect of life has a spiritual component. Spirituality does not have a specific face, name, or denomination.

Religion represents our outward actions in response to our spirituality. Religion is the formal expression of God incarnate that is expressed in relationship with others through education, worship, fellowship, and so forth. Religion has the face of denominations with their various rules, regulations, creeds, rituals, ceremonies, and sacraments.

Internist Christina Puchalski makes similar distinctions between spirituality and religion: "Spirituality is the thing we all have in common; it is the search for the meaning in a person's life. It moves us out of ourselves to other concepts, which could be found in religion, nature, or relationships with others, but it is not exclusive to religion. Spirituality is a much broader concept than religion."

Not everyone makes this distinction. For some individuals, their religion and spirituality are so intertwined that they are virtually one and the same. Dr. Herman Brecher believes that his Jewish faith tradition is synonymous with his spirituality. Other individuals might consider themselves very spiritual but not at all religious. Still others might profess allegiance to a particular denomination yet not feel connected to God or be interested in spiritual issues. Table 1 contrasts religion and spirituality.

Chaplain Rodger Murchison and Dr. Sandra Jamison express con-

TABLE 1. Characteristics Distinguishing Religion and Spirituality

Religion	*Spirituality*
Community focused	Individualistic
Observable, measurable, objective	Less visible and measurable, more subjective
Formal, orthodox, organized	Less formal, less orthodox, less systematic
Behavior oriented, outward practices	Emotionally oriented, inward directed
Authoritarian in terms of behaviors	Not authoritarian, little accountability
Doctrine separating good from evil	Unifying, not doctrine oriented

Taken from H. G. Koenig, et al., (2001) *Handbook of Religion and Health* (New York: Oxford University Press), 18.

cern that some of the current definitions of spirituality are too loose and fail to connect people to God but instead focus on "feeling good" and experiencing a "sense of connectedness" to something without substance.[10] Plante and Sherman, who observe that the sacred is not always part of a spiritual quest for the transcendent, reflect this concern. They contend that "being captivated by a sunset, a sports team, or a political campaign is not intrinsically a spiritual experience simply because one feels connected to something larger than oneself."[11] Emmons and Crumpler, however, believe that ordinary activities can be imbued with spiritual meaning if these activities are linked to God "as is the case for a Buddhist focusing mindfully on sweeping the steps or eating a raisin, a Jew reciting a prayer while washing her hands, or a Catholic who views meal preparation as a sacrament."[12] All those who responded to our questionnaire viewed their spirituality as inextricably linked to a relationship with God.

REFLECTIONS

- How do you define religion? Spirituality?
- Do you believe that there is a difference between religion and spirituality? If so, what is the distinction?
- Is it important to know what your patients believe regarding these two terms?
- In what ways would knowing influence your care?

IMPORTANCE OF SPIRITUALITY AND RELIGIOUS BELIEFS TO DAILY WORK

Every participant identified ways that spirituality and/or religious beliefs influence daily work with patients, co-workers, and the employing agency. Dr. Brecher notes, "Morally and ethically, I try to treat my patients and others as I would like to be treated. This was taught to me religiously and in other ways and probably has the greatest effect on my interpersonal dealings."

Cynthia Poort describes the influence of her beliefs:

I try to approach every situation from a spiritual perspective. I ask myself, in the context of eternity, how important is this issue? What is the spiritually and morally right thing to do? It is amazing how many issues are power struggles or personality conflicts that really don't matter in the long run. I have been able to remain "calm in the eye of the storm" by relying on God and realizing that someone bigger, wiser, and infinite is in control of any situation I may encounter. Gaining wealth, power in the organization, or control over others is not important to me. Being able to minister to people's needs and staying true to my own and the agency's mission, vision, and values are important to me. I can follow a true compass through the morass of life both at work and at home by being rooted in a strong faith and integrity.

Miriam Jacik shares her spirituality and religious practices with colleagues in a very indirect manner.

My desire is that my words and actions bespeak what I believe and try to live on a daily basis. I would never choose to impose my belief system or spirituality upon those with whom I work. My experience has been that most often I find co-workers who have religious and spiritual values similar to my own, and there is a special bonding that occurs between us. We tend to support each other in the ways we minister and provide care to patients. Because there is a trend in our healthcare system to provide more holistic care, employers have become more respectful of the spiritual and religious components of people's lives. Alternative medicine is accepted. Research studies are showing the positive impact of faith and religious beliefs upon the health, healing, and well-being of those who are ill.

These advances, I believe, open up the avenue for providing spiritual care to patients with greater freedom. In my personal experience, I have found that employers have been most respectful and accepting when I provided a spiritual component to the nursing care that I gave to the patients I have served. This is probably because the spiritual care was so integrated with the physical and emotional care that no objection could be posed. The care was truly holistic in nature.

Several respondents spoke of their spirituality being at the heart of their identity and as such being involved in every aspect of life. Evelyn Yapp says, "My spirituality is the hidden force behind my daily activities. My decisions in life and my associations with others are guided by this spiritual foundation that I have developed through years of sacrifice and prayer. When I encounter challenges and difficulties, I naturally implement my abilities to solve problems, and when I am unsure I turn to the Lord and my conscience . . . the voices of reason, understanding, faith, hope, and love." Sister Karen Pozniak, a chaplain and educator, simply states, "It is the core of what I am about."

The importance of prayer was mentioned repeatedly as a way of bringing personal spirituality to bear on daily activities. Joyce Kinstlinger says, "I pray often for patients. I also pray with patients who ask for prayer. I never push my religion on anybody. I routinely give up my worries for a patient to a Higher Power." Dianne Smith echoes a similar sentiment: "I typically pray before I go to work, asking for guidance and wisdom in providing safe care. I'm not one to 'preach,' so I wait for opportunities to talk about my faith. It certainly has helped me deal with the deaths of children. These are rough times, when faith discussions come up with families and co-workers. Most importantly, I believe that my behavior should reflect my faith."

Diane Molitor adds, "Every morning I pray for God to guide me, to walk in his way, and to treat his people the way that he wants me to. He helps me be an honest, compassionate, and caring person to all with whom I come into contact throughout my day." Vicki Germer describes her spirituality as "permeating everything, every day, as I pray for the good of my patients and co-workers. I try to serve others and show them God in some small way. I ask people about their spirituality, and I educate them about how optimum wellness includes a healthy spirituality. I encourage them to grow in this area."

Dr. Julie Steiner reflects that out of her spirituality comes a desire to be as empathetic as possible toward patients as well as employees. "The medical system we deal with is incredibly and unnecessarily complicated. I try to remember that those who are not employed in the system don't fully recognize this. They just want good care whenever they need it. I also try to recognize that my employees are the front line and sometimes take a lot of abuse from patients. I want these employees to know how important they are and that they are appreciated."

Charity Johansson explains that she relies on her spiritual connection to direct professional choices: "When I write the articles that are the most meaningful to me, I can't imagine doing it without prayer. Even when I treat patients, especially with light manual tasks, I often find myself saying to God, 'Let my hands be your hands.' I can't tell you the number of times I have been lost in a technique but made just the right move to help a patient after saying that prayer."

Dr. Michael Parker says his spirituality "influences my commitments of time and energy related to my research, teaching, and service to the community. For example, my decision to serve as the president of the West Alabama Officer's Association was a spiritually based decision related to my calling of helping seniors age successfully. Many of the members are elderly, having served our nation during World War II." Expressing a similar sentiment, Dr. Don Berry feels his spirituality allows him to view "the strong and abiding influences of work, profession, and relationships as a stewardship of life, both in confirming and correcting my actions, attitudes—always seeking to center on the expressions of God's love."

Harriet Coeling describes her efforts to encourage nursing students to think about their own spirituality and to prioritize their lives in a way that allows for a relationship with God. With her co-workers, Harriet credits her own spirituality with making her more willing to offer help and encouragement, to recognize that each of her co-workers is a child of God, and as such is beloved by God. In terms of her own career, her spirituality leads to a sense of peace about advancement: "I recognize that it's really God and not myself who advances my career. It makes me willing to assist others in advancing their careers, again, so they can make God's world a better place, a place like he intended it to be." In discussing the influence of her spirituality toward her employing organization, Harriet says, "I think it helps me be more long-suffering and less judgmental (some at least) toward others whose decisions I don't always agree with."

Chaplain Jeffrey Flowers describes the influence of his spirituality on his daily activities: "I am seen as the religious expert in the hospital. That can be restrictive, as people bring a stereotype to their relationship with me. However, I continue to practice a broader spirituality that seems to draw fellow strugglers into communion. My spiritual practices help me cope with the amount of grief and destruction that I see daily, putting in perspective the things that are meaningful."

Concluding this section dealing with the influence of personal spirituality on life, we hear Dr. Karen Soeken's voice: "I try to keep two verses in mind: 'Establish thou the work of my hands' and 'Whatsoever your task, work heartily as serving the Lord and not men.'" These two Scripture passages provide an adequate summary of the thoughts and feelings of all the respondents.

REFLECTIONS

- How is my work influenced by my spirituality? Does it affect the way I treat others? If so, how? Could I do a better job of integrating my spiritual beliefs into my daily activities?
- Is prayer part of my daily routine?
- Am I comfortable discussing spirituality with others in a nonthreatening manner?
- Is spirituality something that I keep to myself?
- In what ways would the healthcare environment be different if everyone lived his or her spirituality?

In this chapter, we listened to the voices of healthcare professionals describe God's call to them to pursue a life of service. We heard them relate how they have responded to that call and how the call to serve has deepened and strengthened over time. We listened as they explained the ways their spirituality is expressed in the caregiving process. We explored the common path of healthcare and ministry and examined the characteristics of a ministering person.

In the next chapter, we continue our journey by examining the state of the current healthcare system and how the system influences spiritual expression among healthcare professionals.

[2]

The State of the Current Healthcare System

The demands on caregivers to keep up with breakthroughs and setbacks, with economic forecasts and paperwork requirements, with "code blues" and needlestick precautions, with fast-moving gurneys and insurer limits are colossal. And I'm afraid that the things that imbue our patients' lives with meaning—the values, fears, and sources of solace that immediately come to mind when one's health is threatened—frequently get disregarded in this whirlwind of change.

—Dr. Herbert Benson, *Timeless Healing*

Our healthcare system is in crisis. Many would identify it as an economic crisis, with the focus on profit making as a detriment to care, and indeed this focus is a major issue. But the crisis is broader and deeper than the for-profit model of healthcare would suggest. It is a true identity crisis and may ultimately be a spiritual one.

In the midst of trying to balance the competing demands that swirl around healthcare providers, some may lose sight of their ministry and their call to be healers. They may pull away from patients and insulate themselves against the pain that calls out to them from patients and families. This interpersonal distance only increases the healthcare providers' sense of discontent and intensifies their own pain. They may wonder, Is this all there is? I didn't become a doctor, nurse, social worker, or therapist to deal with insurance companies that want to limit care. I didn't enter this field to feel like I was on a treadmill every day just trying to do the basic minimum for my patients.

These are questions of meaning and purpose: What is the meaning of my life? What is the meaning of my profession? And, do I make a difference? Sometimes these questions lead to such profound disillusionment that the healthcare provider chooses either to walk away, as nurses have done in droves, or to push feelings of discontent out of awareness and settle for providing care that is less than satisfactory.[1]

There is an epidemic of low staff morale and burnout in medicine and nursing, making it difficult to hire and retain staff and affecting the quality of patient care.[2] Staff turnover is as high as 40 percent per year in some hospitals. Malpractice insurance rates are rising out of sight because of increasing litigation, due at least in part to poor doctor-patient relationships and patient dissatisfaction with the limited biotechnological care that they are receiving.[3]

What is missing in the doctor-patient relationship? Lack of trust, we think, is one factor. A trusting relationship exists between doctor and patient when the doctor respects the patient as a unique individual and addresses the patient as a whole person—including body, mind, social relationships, and spirit. When that is the case, litigation almost never occurs. Even if mistakes are made, the patient is usually willing to forgive the physician to preserve the relationship. Physicians, too, get more out of their job as providers when they deliver care in this way.

One reason that whole-person care is becoming less and less common today is the loss of a sense of ministry or spiritual "calling" among health professionals. There is evidence that having a sense of calling may influence staff morale, productivity, sick days, and burnout rates among healthcare workers.[4] Consequently, addressing the spiritual needs of hospital staff may need to become a priority.[5] Training health professionals to integrate spirituality into patient care may help them recognize, develop, and value their own spirituality, their sense of calling, and the satisfaction they experience with their work.

IMPACT OF THE WORK ENVIRONMENT

In our interviews, we asked participants questions about the healthcare system. First, we wanted to know if participants believed that the current healthcare system had an impact on their own spirituality. Second, we asked whether or not the healthcare workplace had the potential to be a spiritual environment. Third, we inquired about ways that participants contribute to the spiritual environment of the healthcare workplace. Fourth, we asked whether participants believed that an intangible such as a spiritual environment affects employee retention. Fifth and last, we provided a list of concepts that are identified in the literature as necessary for a spiritual work environment and asked each participant to prioritize these concepts and comment on the top three.

Although many of our participants asserted that the current healthcare system has a negative impact on their personal spirituality, there were a few individuals who believed that the healthcare system actually strengthened their own spirituality, and one nurse stated that the healthcare system had no impact on her spirituality. Those who identified a negative impact focused on insurance restrictions, lack of or inadequate healthcare coverage for some patients, the burden of navigating a maze of bureaucratic requirements, an overly litigious society prone to legal suits, the deterioration of the relationship between patients and healthcare providers, and a culture that depersonalizes patients. Those who said the healthcare system actually strengthened their spirituality identified the same problems but concluded that these problems made them more dependent on prayer and a vital relationship to God. There were also a few participants who were neutral in their responses.

Negative impact. Physician Jack Hasson declares, "Negative factors such as lack of funding for healthcare and medications for patients and the amount of 'red tape' in medical practice are barriers to the mission of caring for our patients. This requires us to spend time on issues that lessen the time we would like to spend on spiritual issues with patients, staff, and others." Retired oncologist Alton Lightsey finds that "the increased demand for justification and documentation compete for time and energy to care for patients, families, and colleagues." In a similar vein, Joanne Smith, a nursing administrator, adds, "The healthcare system challenges my spirituality every day as I struggle with what needs to be done for a patient and what insurance and various regulations say I can do. The patient does not always come out a winner in this struggle."

Mitroff and Denton identify the importance of shared values of service as a foundation for creating a spiritual work environment.[6] Commenting on the importance of values from a nursing perspective, Nancy Hines notes:

The current healthcare system often challenges my spirituality. For instance, I am challenged to make sure I care for people as valued individuals and not as a way to make money. I have to look for ways to build caring into every interaction. Clearly the work environment can either promote caring or destroy it through the values that are explicit as well as implicit in the culture of the workplace. I contribute by challenging values, by asking tough questions, and by following through on issues, problems, and ideas. Sometimes I feel as though I am a lone voice arguing for a more caring and spiritual approach to problems. I get especially concerned when I see an attitude of "planned neglect" color the care provided to the debilitated elderly. It seems as if the conclusion that "This is Mr. Smith's time to die" is arrived at much too easily, with little respect or caring directed toward that individual. It's almost as if we are throwing people away.

Nancy is not alone in her disdain for the ever-present focus on the bottom line. Vicki Germer, a psychiatric nurse, complains, "I am so frustrated by the current healthcare system; everything seems to be about money, and there is so much more that we should think about, like doing our best to help patients and families dealing with psychiatric problems."

Mohrmann contends that the practice of medicine has as its central metaphor the image of the healthcare provider as a minister: "We who minister to those who suffer are called to love them, and this means that we are to give ourselves—our knowledge, our time, our passion, our strength—without stint."[7] Increasingly, this image is challenged by a system that demands more from its practitioners and allows far less time for patients.

Dr. Bernita Taylor poignantly laments the change in the doctor-patient relationship: "The doctor-patient relationship used to be almost sacred—it was on a higher plane. Now it is more a business relationship. The doctor is a merchant and the patient is a consumer. In the process, we have lost something very precious." Dr. Tom Grace, also focusing on the doctor-patient relationship, says, "As medicine becomes more of a business, it is absolutely essential that 'good' people stay in medicine. The personal relationship is critical, and we need to take the extra step to make sure that it happens."

The practice of medicine has as its central metaphor the image of the healthcare provider as a minister: "We who minister to those who suffer are called to love them, and this means that we are to give ourselves—our knowledge, our time, our passion, our strength—without stint."

Of course, other healthcare professionals feel the challenges to a healing relationship as well. Harriet Coeling, a nurse faculty member, describes the work environment of nurses as one that diminishes who they are and what they can contribute to the nurse-patient relationship.

I think the main reasons nurses leave a job situation or leave nursing completely are lack of respect from those they work for and with whom they interact, a lack of appreciation for what they do, and the unreasonable work conditions they face. I think these factors come from a desire to enhance profits and/or a desire to make oneself appear better than others (nurses). So I think that if more people in the organization could see the image of God in each worker and treat each person with the dignity and respect due to God himself (in a more spiritual environment), we could indeed prevent so many nurses from leaving nursing.

Dr. Sandra Jamison, a retired nursing professor, finds the state of the healthcare system very discouraging because it is so market driven. She decries the depersonalization of patients and caregivers alike: "The heart of nursing is the person, and today the person is viewed as just another market commodity." On a similar note, Dr. Sagrid Eleanor Edman, retired nursing dean of Bethel College, observes, "The current health-care system makes me angry. I am frustrated because I am sure that so many patients are not getting their needs met. Currently I am working with parish nurses, and I really emphasize the advocacy role of the parish nurse—someone needs to speak up for the patient and make sure that needs are met!"

Even hospital chaplains feel the constraints of less time available for developing a healing relationship. Jeffrey Flowers observes, "We are asked to be more global, experts in all religious expressions to ensure that all people have their needs met. We are also asked to do more with less, to build faster relationships, which, of course, will be less meaning-ful. People move through the system so quickly it is hard to know them."

Another nurse, Miriam Jacik, provides a scathing evaluation of the current healthcare system:

Presently our healthcare system endorses healthcare delivery that is fast paced, impersonal, and by all means cost saving. The patient is very often lost in the process. In the name of efficiency, we have sacrificed personhood. In the name of progress, we have tread upon ethical and moral values. To remain involved in healthcare, as we presently know it, requires that the care provider have a spiri-tuality and set of personal religious values that are strong enough to meet the challenges of the times. The recipients of our care need to find caregivers who are persons of integrity with moral values and principles that direct their lives. I believe that spirituality must be alive and ever deepening in my life and in the lives of all dedicated healthcare providers.

Sometimes the rules that govern "professional" practice get in the way of spirituality. Charity Johansson elaborates: "The constraints of the healthcare system make it more challenging to work as a whole being, honoring the spiritual in ourselves and our patients. For example, if a dying patient asks me to pray with her, I will. But then to be ethical, do I track the minutes of prayer and subtract them from the physical ther-apy time? I sometimes feel a little shaky stepping outside traditional practice. There's such a move for evidence-based practice, but the assumptions underlying evidence-based practice don't allow much role for spirit. It's so man-made."

Positive impact. Eileen Altenhofer, a parish nurse, agrees that the current healthcare system is very hard for everyone to cope with—it is complicated, expensive, and often inaccessible. However, she says, "It influences my spirituality by making me feel I need to pray more to have patience and perseverance." Reflecting a similar position, Genie Ford adds, "The healthcare system makes me pray. There are many issues for concern, such as the lack of healthcare for everyone and the nursing shortage. These issues are so overwhelming, but the one thing that I can consistently do is to pray."

Harriet Coeling concurs:

The stresses of the current system make me more aware of my need to maintain my relationship with God and to draw upon him for the strength and guidance I need to get through each day. Healthcare today is so complex that I find I need a personal focus to guide my decisions and to make wise ones. I see the whole world as a spiritual environment, a place that draws me into deeper relationship with God. I think both peaceful and stressful places can draw me closer to God, although they do so in different ways.

From the perspective of an occupational therapist, Jay Brashear explains the impact of the healthcare system on his spirituality.

When I felt initially called to be an occupational therapist, I believed that I would be a really good OT. Now I recognize that I am probably an average clinician. But I can see that the reason God wants me in this profession is for what I contribute spiritually. God has given me the ability to think outside of the box, to call a spade a spade, and an overwhelming desire, despite today's inadequate healthcare system, to make patients feel unique and loved and not just another case. I believe that the current healthcare system does not offer people reasonable options for getting well. As a system it is failing. As a clinician, I hope that my prayers for a patient plus my call to be with them will give them something that they really need, and that is full healing.

Neutral impact. Diane Molitor, a nurse, explains her perspective: "The current healthcare system does not influence my spirituality; my spirituality influences how I react in the current healthcare system. My spirituality makes me more aware of the importance of being honest and sincere with others and exercising the Golden Rule—that is, treating others as I would like to be treated. I recognize how important it is to be compassionate and caring not only to patients and their families but to co-workers as well."

Dee Brooks, another nurse, responds:

I am not sure if the system influences my spirituality. I think we should be more aware of and provide for a patient and family's spiritual needs, and that I just may have been called to see that this happens as part of my total care for these people. A hospital workplace is a place where you see people's vulnerabilities in a time of stress—this can include co-workers as well as patients and families. When you allow the peace of Christ to shine through via calmness, quiet, listening, doing caring acts, and touching, this is often felt by those around you, and it spreads.

Most who work with me know my religious convictions and appreciate who I am because of them. I am not shy about asking a person's religious practice and if I can help in any way to see their needs are met while in the hospital. If asked to pray, I am there. Hopefully, through my actions those around me who are not as comfortable with these issues or had not considered the workplace a spiritual environment can learn from me how to incorporate spirituality in their work and be comfortable with it.

REFLECTIONS

- In what ways does the current healthcare system have an impact on your own spirituality?
- In what ways does the culture of the healthcare system affect your ability to act as a ministering person?
- Think about a recent interaction with a patient, family, or colleague, from which you walked away feeling good about what occurred. How did your spirituality influence that interaction?

🕮 Think about a recent interaction with a patient, family, or colleague from which you walked away feeling dissatisfied with how you handled that interaction. Describe what you would have liked the out come to be. In what ways would your spirituality have brought about the desired outcome?

THE HEALTHCARE SYSTEM:
A SPIRITUAL ENVIRONMENT

We asked in what ways the healthcare workplace is a spiritual environment. Most of our respondents talked about the power of individual example to shape, influence, and create such an environment. Some identified the importance of externals, such as a pleasing décor and the availability of quiet, private spaces within the healthcare facility. Others discussed the influence of leadership in the creation of a spiritual culture. One nurse, Margie Schmier, told us that the only workplace that she believed was spiritual was that of hospice, with its focus on end-of-life spiritual issues.

Let's listen to the voices of the participants.

According to nurse Genie Ford, the core activity of caring makes the healthcare system a spiritual workplace: "If you look at life as a spiritual journey, then your workplace will naturally be a place where spirituality can be practiced. Caring for people is a spiritual endeavor."

Chaplain Jeffrey Flowers also comments on the significance of caring relationships in healthcare: "So much time is spent in a workplace with important relationships being nurtured, it seems impossible that it would not be a spiritual environment. Of course, it can also be a negative spiritual environment if people feel threatened or suppressed in their workplace. In order to be productive, it seems that one must find the ability to be at ease with one's spirit, to find meaning and purpose in what one does."

Dr. Sagrid Eleanor Edman believes that the commitment of individuals to integration of faith into everything makes the workplace a spiritual environment.

Dr. Jack Hasson recognizes "that the workplace is shaped by those that enter it—many have different and often foreign approaches to spirituality. We need to lead by our personal examples of spiritual approaches to what we do, but be open to others and their approaches, which work for them—this is especially true for patients when they are ill and stressed."

In discussing the influence of the external factors, Eileen Altenhofer points out, "A workplace can be spiritual by making the environment more peaceful, quieter, pleasant to view, and perhaps most importantly, by the smiles on the faces of the staff." Adding to this, Charity Johansson suggests, "I think any workplace that provides some quiet private space begins to provide a spiritual environment. I still need some privacy for my prayer, and I need to be in environments that are beautiful—visually, auditorally, and tactilely. Such environments feed my soul and help sustain my spirit. In the same way, allowing for enjoyable experiences promotes spiritual being."

Dr. Karen Soeken comments that in order for the workplace to be a spiritual environment, it must be a place of growth, encouragement, and development of talents and abilities with a "peaceful yet energetic ambience."

Mitroff and Denton contend that the leadership of an organization plays a critical role in creating a spiritual environment: "No organization can survive for long without spirituality and soul. . . . We need to integrate spirituality into management. We must find ways of managing spirituality without separating it from other elements of management."[8]

Nancy Shoemaker, a psychiatric nurse, makes similar observations: "All workplaces have an atmosphere or culture. When the leadership staff recognize the importance of spirituality and demonstrate spiritual values—respect for patients and staff alike, honesty, integrity, hope—not only do staff feel valued, but there is ongoing hope for patients to improve."

Working in the home environment gives Jay Brashear a slightly different perspective: "If the workplace is the patient's home, then it is absolutely a spiritual

> "No organization can survive for long without spirituality and soul. . . . We need to integrate spirituality into management. We must examine ways of managing spirituality without separating it from the other elements of management."

environment. This is where the patient has been accustomed to practicing very personal activities such as getting cleaned and dressed, which
are things that most people are able to do in their own home. When
someone is unable to do something that everyone else can do in their
own homes, then the home becomes the ground on which they want
to be healed—physically and spiritually."

Miriam Jacik provides a summary of what is essential for the workplace to be a spiritual environment:

*It is necessary for the supervisory staff as well as the care providers within the envi-
ronment to be persons of integrity with high moral standards and values and have
lives that are directed by spiritual principles. Such an environment will be graced
by the personal gifts of each caregiver. Collectively they will create an atmosphere
of love, caring, goodness, and peace that can't help but emanate from them and
touch the lives of all the patients who enter that environment. When a spirit of
ministry, as opposed to mere job performance, exists, persons with needs of any
kind who enter that environment will have their needs more adequately met.*

*However, a work environment that is contaminated by standards of greed, cor-
ruption, dishonesty, and power-seeking that filter down from the level of upper
management is hard pressed to have spirituality develop and flourish to any real
degree. Evil and a pervading lack of morality can corrupt a whole organization,
making it very difficult for goodness, justice, and other spiritual values to exist.
Persons of faith, morals, and spiritual practice can individually and collectively
affect their work environment, rendering it a spiritual environment. It takes the
personal conviction that the way one lives one's life can affect in a positive way
those around oneself.*

*I believe this and trust that my spirituality and religious convictions do make
a difference in my work environment and in the lives of those I serve in ministry.
Being true to what I believe and having it be reflected in my choices and actions
contribute to the environment in which I work. Finding myself in an environment that is not life-giving and perhaps corrupt challenges me to endeavor to be
a change agent in some way. If I find that efforts at bringing goodness, rightness,
truth, and integrity to an environment are futile, this is an indication to me that
I must leave the environment.*

REFLECTIONS

- In what ways is your work environment a spiritual one?
- What factors support and/or hinder your work environment from being a spiritual one?
- How would you rate the importance of external factors, such as décor and provision of quiet spaces for prayer and contemplation, in the creation of a spiritual work environment? How important are individual internal factors such as commitment to caring and ministry in creating a spiritual environment?
- What is the role of leadership in creating and communicating a spiritual culture in the workplace?

INDIVIDUAL CONTRIBUTIONS
TO THE CREATION OF A SPIRITUAL
ENVIRONMENT

A common theme of caring and serving others ran through our participants' responses to the question, "In what ways are you able to contribute to the spiritual environment of your workplace?"

When a spirit of ministry, as opposed to mere job performance, exists, persons with needs of any kind who enter that environment will have their needs more adequately met. Often, however, a work environment that is contaminated by standards of greed, corruption, dishonesty, and power-seeking that filter down from the level of upper management can be hard pressed to have spirituality develop and flourish to any real degree.

Dr. Jack Hasson says, "My contribution to the spirituality of the work environment is by reflecting love, caring, and concern for my fellow workers and patients in a sincere and genuine manner." Dr. Bernita Taylor takes a similar approach: "I make sure to acknowledge the importance of other workers in our office and how we all depend on one another to get the job done. It is so important to be supportive to co-workers who are experiencing stressful times."

Harriet Coeling elaborates:

In my organization, I try to represent God's love to others with the hopes that some might come closer to God through this effort, and I try to help others see my interpretation of how God is active in my life and helps me in so many ways.

I share with others in the hope that others might better understand how God wants to be recognized by them as being active in their lives. I try to behave in a loving, patient, joyful manner so that I can contribute to making the workplace a more spiritually healthy place in which to work.

Eileen Altenhofer shares her efforts to make the external environment more spiritual, as well as her volunteer caring efforts that go above and beyond the call to serve others: "In my current parish nurse role, I try to incorporate spiritual components into displays. For example, I prepare a monthly bulletin board highlighting a particular resource theme. There is always a poem, a Bible verse, or an uplifting thought related to the theme that is incorporated into the bulletin board. I also volunteer at Highline Hospital, where I research health topics in the Planetree Library. I prepare information packets for hospital patients at their request, answering questions about their particular illness."

Patricia Camp, a nurse, laments:

There are things that I see in the hospital environment that detract greatly from it being a spiritual atmosphere. Valuing and respecting others is spiritual and is expressed in many different ways. When I hear caregivers use foul language and or engage in any type of "verbal abuse of patients," the atmosphere is certainly not a spiritual one. I also believe that the appearance of the healthcare professional also contributes to or takes away from a spiritual environment. Uniforms should always be neat, clean, and professional in appearance. This outward sign is a reflection of how individual practitioners value their profession as well as how they value and respect patients.

Vicki Germer, a psychiatric nurse, identifies the responsibility of the individual for contributing to the spiritual environment: "I engage in positive conversations that focus on the good in people and situations. I also contribute through prayer, sometimes my own silent prayer and at other times shared prayer, through music, and through a positive, caring attitude."

Dr. Tom Grace also highlights the importance of personal prayer as a contribution to making the work environment a spiritual one: "I pray for my patients before surgery, and many times they ask me to join them in prayer, which I always do. Prayer is also important for the staff that I work with, so I also pray for them."

Dr. Karen Soeken identifies intrinsic qualities that contribute to spirituality, such as being a person of integrity, showing respect for others, being a good listener, and being someone who others can come to without feeling judged or demeaned. She also highlights the importance of extrinsic factors such as the atmosphere of her office—the art on the walls and the desk, as well as the music that she has playing. All these factors contribute to a spiritual environment.

Kelly Preston, the former congregational health program coordinator for the Ingalls Center for Pastoral Ministries, believes that the presence of a parish nurse program contributes to the spiritual environment of the facility. The fact that a healthcare institution supports such a program is recognition of the important relationship between faith and health.

A home care nurse, Karen McCauley, believes that the presence of nurture and support to others is foundational to a spiritual workplace.

I think it is important for nurses to get together to discuss their concerns and to support one another. Sometimes meetings like this can be very negative; however, they also have the potential for producing positive ideas and generating support for the team. From a personal perspective, I believe I contribute to a spiritual environment by helping others in any way that I can. I try to always be optimistic; it helps me cope with situations that are beyond my control. Also, I believe that being negative seems to draw forth more negativity from others and really has a detrimental impact on the whole environment. The Prayer of St. Francis is my favorite; I say it every day and make a conscious effort to follow it.

> *Lord, make me an instrument of Thy peace.*
> *Where there is hatred, let me sow love.*
> *Where there is injury, pardon.*
> *Where there is doubt, faith.*
> *Where there is despair, hope.*
> *Where there is darkness, light.*
> *Where there is sadness, joy.*

> *O Divine Master,*
> *Grant that I may not so much seek to be consoled, as to console;*
> *To be understood, as to understand,*
> *To be loved, as to love;*
> *For it is in giving that we receive,*
> *It is in pardoning that we are pardoned,*
> *And it is in dying that we are born to eternal life.*

Dr. Christina Puchalski believes that "it is essential that we respect the beliefs of others and that we focus our understanding on the core values rather than the differences of each religion. We would find that we have much more in common than is different. If the workplace is to be spiritual, it is essential that people feel cared for, supported, respected, and loved."

Her own efforts are directed not just to her work environment at George Washington University School of Medicine but toward system-wide changes. She founded and directs the George Washington Institute for Spirituality and Health, a university-based organization working toward a more compassionate system of healthcare. The institute has proposed the following changes:

PHYSICIANS AND OTHER HEALTHCARE PROVIDERS WILL:

1. Recognize and accept that they are entrusted with the care of:
 • *the physical,*
 • *the emotional,*
 • *the social,*
 • *and the spiritual aspects of their patients in all phases of*
  patients' lives;
2. Support patients in their suffering and in the midst of existential pain;
3. Address spiritual values and beliefs as part of the routine medical
history;
4. Form collaborative partnerships with chaplains, clergy, and other spiritual
care providers; and
5. Recognize that their own spirituality plays a key role in their professional
lives and affects how they interact with their patients and colleagues.

MEDICINE AND HEALTHCARE WILL INCLUDE:

1. A field of spirituality and health whereby physicians and other health-care providers can further their academic and professional interests in order to improve the care of patients;

2. An increased amount of scholarly research by a variety of disciplines on the roles of spirituality and health;

3. Health administrators and healthcare policymakers who recognize the importance of spirituality in healthcare; and

4. Healthcare training programs in spirituality and health that span all disciplines.

SOCIETAL CHANGES:

1. A recognition of the role of spirituality in healthcare, and particularly in chronic illness and end-of-life care; and

2. An increased awareness by and an empowering of the nonmedical public regarding the role of spirituality, particularly in chronic illness and end-of-life care.

—Taken from www.gwish.org/id17.htm

REFLECTIONS

- What do you bring to the healthcare workplace that contributes to a positive spirituality?
- How do you live out your spirituality in the workplace?
- Consider the problems that you encounter at work—how would spirituality influence the solutions to these problems?

SPIRITUALITY AND EMPLOYEE RETENTION

In a study reported by Trott, spiritual well-being was evaluated among 184 workers at a Fortune 100 engineering-construction organization.[9] The sample demonstrated a moderately high level of spiritual well-being as well as significantly positive relationships between spiritual well-being and perceptions of organizational openness, general self-efficacy, and normative and affective organizational commitment.

Additionally, a significant inverse relationship was found between spiritual well-being and commitment to staying in the job. Although there are no similar studies that examine the healthcare environment, the responses of our participants seem to indicate that Trott's findings might be generalizable to the healthcare system. When we asked participants whether an intangible such as spirituality could effect employee retention, we received overwhelming affirmation to this suggestion.

Charity Johansson responded, "I think the degree to which an employer environment acknowledges the value of and promotes the health of the whole person—body, spirit, and soul—including the intellect, emotions, and imagination—strongly affects retention. There will always be some turnover, which isn't necessarily a bad thing. But often people leave because something is moving in or out of balance."

Surgeon Tom Grace believes that an environment where employees feel supported and valued for their contributions to a culture of care produces high morale and low turnover. Expressing a similar viewpoint, physician Jack Hasson says, "Employee retention is certainly positively impacted by an enjoyable work environment where spiritual matters are experienced as a natural concern. This allows workers to feel at home and to look forward to work every day, knowing they are working for a greater good. In such an environment, even the stressor of increased work and slightly less compensation will not be viewed in such a negative fashion as to lead to employee turnover."

In total agreement, psychiatric nurse Nancy Shoemaker believes "the supportive culture resulting from a spiritual environment is very instrumental in employee satisfaction and retention. Staff such as myself will work under adverse conditions with very difficult patients when there is a shared belief system that values each individual as a precious human being."

Kelly Preston comments that sometimes there is a pull between pay and benefits versus a spiritual culture as factors influencing retention: "I do believe that a spiritual environment influences retention; however, sometimes money can be a driving force for many nurses who may be single parents and will leave a position for another where pay and benefits are better. Yet here at Baptist Health System, we have many employees who have been here more than thirty years! Employees say that the mission of the hospital to the provision of pastoral care is the reason for their longevity."

Feeling loved and cared about are not only important for patients but for healthcare providers as well. Eileen Altenhofer says, "I believe staff is more likely to stay because spiritual components in an environment contribute to a feeling of calmness and being cared for. Happier patients result in the staff feeling more satisfied with their delivery of care."

Diane Molitor, a nurse, adds, "In a true spiritual environment, you would see employee retention. People don't tend to run away from warmth, caring, honesty, or a relaxed environment where they can be themselves."

Dr. Bernita Taylor also supports the view that employees prefer to remain in a work environment where they are loved and respected.

Miriam Jacik reflects on her nursing experience:

I believe that a spiritual environment is a felt experience for those who work in it and has positive aspects that are perceived by caregivers. A spiritual environment, even though it may be wrought with busyness, stress, or difficult situations, is different and is felt to be different by those working in it. There is a sense of God-given strength, peace, and goodness pervading the whole environment. This allows one to balance the negative factors such as stress and busyness against existing factors that are positive.

This, I believe, draws caregivers to want to be in such an environment, to decrease turnover, and to increase retention. In the thirty years that I have practiced nursing, I have found that a chaotic work environment with no positive aspects like a spiritual environment affords will most likely lead to frequent staff burnout and a high rate of staff turnover.

Chaplain Jeffrey Flowers's observations conclude this section: "It is clear that where people are happy, they are more productive, and when they feel that what they do has purpose, they will do it with greater pride. These are spiritual words and concepts. Also, a spiritual community cares for one another. Employees who feel cared for are more likely to be loyal and to stay."

REFLECTIONS

ᘉ Do you believe that a spiritual work environment influences employee retention and turnover? If so, in what ways does this occur?

ᘉ Think about employee retention and turnover in your place of work. How is spirituality an influencing factor?

ᘉ What factors would make you stay or leave a place of employment? Have you ever left a position because the environment was not spiritual? What was it like?

NECESSARY COMPONENTS OF A SPIRITUAL WORKPLACE

We identified fourteen concepts from the literature focusing on spirituality in the workplace, and we asked participants to prioritize the top three and comment on why these concepts were most important. The concepts included: (1) meaningful work; (2) purposeful activity;[10] (3) affirmation; (4) interconnectedness and relationships;[11] (5) shared values; (6) concern for ethical and moral dilemmas; (7) open communication; (8) reasonable expectations regarding productivity standards, paperwork requirements, and other responsibilities;[12] (9) support for spiritual care for patients and families;[13] (10) authenticity; (11) awareness; (12) congruency;[14] (13) a focus on the patient; and (14) a sense of vocation.[15]

Table 2 shows the ranking of each of the top three concepts.

Meaningful work was ranked as the most important concept by thirteen of the participants; interconnectedness and relationships was ranked second in importance by twelve of the participants; and shared values was ranked third in importance by seven of the participants.

Let's listen to what participants told us regarding the importance of these concepts.

Meaningful Work

Everyone who ranked meaningful work as the most important component in a spiritual environment had similar comments. Othelia Lee, a social work professor, exclaims, "I feel passionate about what I do!" Dr.

TABLE 2. Ranking of Importance of Fourteen Spiritual Concepts

Spiritual Concept	1st-Place Ranking	2nd-Place Ranking	3rd-Place Ranking	Total Weighted Score‡
Meaningful work	13	5	1	50★
Purposeful activity	3	3	–	15
Affirmation	–	3	5	11
Interconnectedness	4	12	5	41★★
Shared values	3	2	7	20
Ethical and moral concern		3	4	10
Open communication	2	7	5	25
Focus on patient	11	2	2	39★★★
Reasonable work expectations		3	6	12
Open support for spiritual care	5	2	2	21
Authenticity	1	2	2	9
Awareness	1	–	–	3
Congruency	–	–	–	–
Sense of vocation	3	1	–	11

‡ The first place votes were given three points, the second place votes received two points, and the third place votes received one point. A total was obtained for each spiritual concept.

★ Most important concept ★★ Second most important concept ★★★ Third most important concept

Michael Parker, a gerontology specialist, espouses a similar view: "A sense of calling provides and fosters contagious passion." Joyce Kinstlinger, a community resource counselor. agrees: "You've got to want to make a difference and put your heart into what you are doing with patients and colleagues." Cynthia Poort, a nurse involved in mental health treatment, asserts, "It is essential that work impacts your life and the lives of others—otherwise why do it?" Sister Karen Pozniak concurs: "Unless work is meaningful, it is hard to do it. When work is meaningful, it is carried out with the heart and not willpower." Dr. Daniel Ober believes that "work must have meaning to give us a sense of who and what we are." Nurse Genie Ford adds, "One has to perceive that what one is doing is important to the overall mission of the organization, whether it is being on the janitorial staff or the management team."

Interconnectedness and Relationships

Many participants commented on the significance of interconnectedness and relationships with God, with patients, and with colleagues.

Sandra Brown, a nurse practitioner, speaks about the nurse–patient relationship: "It is through relationships that patients find meaning in their circumstances and in their suffering. The nurse–patient relationship is bound by a sacred trust that nurses will always seek to meet their patients' needs. This requires the nurse to enter the patient's presence with the intent to connect in a meaningful and spiritual way."

Carol Story, also commenting on the importance of relationships, believes, "When all is said and done, if people are not connected to one another either by values, dreams, goals, faith, or work, life has little meaning, and a deep sense of loss exists."

Focus on Patient

The focus on the patient was chosen as the third most important concept. The comments of many of the nurse participants were similar. Karen McCauley states, "My work is the patient and how the patient is treated involves my spirituality." Diane Molitor emphasizes the importance of a focus on the patient, "The patient is the reason for our work." Eileen Altenhofer explains, "If we focus on the patient, we become less task oriented. This is a very tall order during the current nursing shortage and short hospital stays of patients. However if we take the extra step of imparting to the patient that we really care how they feel and how they are progressing, it contributes to their healing and ultimately there is a better outcome. And finally, Dr. Gunnar Christiansen states, "A spiritual environment will not develop unless the patient comes first. In a medical office or a hospital, the purpose in utilizing our God given gifts is to give care for others as persons. Unless we primarily put our focus on our patients, it is likely that we will focus only on their disease."

REFLECTIONS

ᘒ How would you prioritize the fourteen concepts?

ᘒ How do you see these concepts operationalized where you work?

ᘒ How would you like to see these concepts operationalized? Identify one action that you could take to make this happen.

This chapter has reviewed the spiritual crisis of the healthcare system. We have examined the pressures and demands on healthcare professionals to do more with less and to meet unreasonable demands for documentation and for regulatory compliance. We have heard the voices of nurses, doctors, therapists, chaplains, social workers, and others describe the impact that the healthcare system has on their own spirituality as well as their conclusions regarding the potential of the healthcare system to be a spiritual environment. They have also shared their own stories of how they continually strive to make the healthcare system what it should be, a healing and ministering environment. We have listened to their voices affirming that an environment lacking in spirituality has difficulty holding onto employees. And last, we hear these same healthcare providers telling us that it is ultimately important that their work be meaningful and structured around relationships and interconnectedness with patients, families, and colleagues and bound together by shared values.

Before continuing with chapter 3, which takes us to the next step and suggests what the ideal healthcare system might look like, let's listen to one more voice, that of Chaplain Robb Small: "The healthcare system needs more communication and much less emotional abuse of its employees. There needs to be greater effort to understand the balance between the financial margin and the spiritual mission. Success and financial tails wag the dog. I would like to see some of this turned around. I would like to see the leadership of institutions realize that as long as the focus is upside-down, work will be a painful struggle instead of a joyful service that one can be excited to get up each morning looking forward to the day."

[3]

Envisioning the Ideal

As healers we have to receive the stories of our fellow human beings with compassionate hearts, hearts that do not judge or condemn but recognize boundaries within which the often painful past can be revealed and the search for a new life can find a start.

—Henri Nouwen, *Ministry and Spirituality*

What do healthcare professionals think is necessary to make the environment "spiritually healthy"? What would an ideal healthcare environment look like? How would we function in such an environment? Is there any existing healthcare system that comes close to the ideal? Is the hope for a healthcare system that embraces the spirit of all just a fanciful notion, or could it be a reality?

This chapter describes a vision for such a healthcare system, examines how the roles of healthcare providers would operate in such a system, elaborates on the ways patients and families would benefit from it, and presents examples of healthcare systems that embody aspects of the vision.

WHAT HEALTHCARE PROFESSIONALS WANT

We asked participants, "What would you like to see done in the workplace that supports your personal efforts at bringing spirituality into healthcare?" The responses reflected a number of common concerns, but the primary theme was a need for leadership that embodies spiritual values, supports spiritual care for patients and families, and provides spiritual support for the caregiver. The comments of our respondents demonstrate their recognition of the power of one person to make a difference to a patient, a group, and even a culture. Many expressed a strong desire for more kindness, compassion, acceptance of differences—including religious differences—and better communication.

Beyond these behaviors, participants recognized that what is needed is a system change of such magnitude that it would require focused intention, long-term commitment, and an acceptance of spiritual values that cherishes individuals and recognizes the significance of the work done by care providers. We have organized the text in this chapter to first examine the leadership issues. Then we address the changes needed to provide support for the spiritual care of patients. Last, we address suggestions for supporting the spirituality of the healthcare provider. In addition to these areas of focus, we include two responses that reflect totally different perspectives on the question, "What would you like to see done in the workplace that supports your personal efforts at bringing spirituality into healthcare?"

Leadership Issues

Quite a few of our participants commented on the importance of leadership in changing the healthcare culture. Dr. Gunnar Christiansen says, "The development of an environment in the workplace that fosters spiritual growth is dependent on the example of one employee for another and particularly by those in management. This will not come out by regulations or suggestions. It will occur only through demonstration of love for one another, which requires appreciation of each person and being sensitive to his or her needs and feelings."

Patricia Camp contends that the value of spiritual care must be not

The development of an environment in the workplace that fosters spiritual growth is dependent on the example of one employee for another and particularly by those in management. This will not come out by regulations or suggestions. It will only occur through demonstration of love for one another, which requires appreciation of each person and being sensitive to his or her needs and feelings.
—Dr. Gunnar Christiansen

only recognized but required by hospital administrators if this is to become a reality. In full agreement, Dr. Karen Soeken observes, "It is essential for management to have spiritual values. It is too bad it's not a job requirement for management level!"

From the perspective of a healthcare administrator, Martha Loveland makes several very specific suggestions for the leadership of a healthcare organization.

I'd like to see corporate objectives set which are based on reasonable resources. Workload data should be shared/published so senior managers would have an objective base for making resource allocation decisions. I'd like all levels of senior management to participate in every level of employment in the company. This would assist upper management to more accurately perceive, understand, and then manage the human issues that relate to the job. The employee must be valued and the employee must know he or she is valued in every feasible way. I'd like to see family needs recognized better with flexible scheduling, paid paternity leave, more paid vacation, and a workday not to exceed eight hours. Single parenting and blended families exert extreme pressure on the whole family in trying to cope with communication and decision issues. The employee must be understood as having other interests and responsibilities beyond the work place.

REFLECTIONS

- In what ways does the leadership of your healthcare organization support spiritual care? Spiritual well-being of employees?
- What would you like management to do to make your workplace environment more spiritually supportive to patients, families, and caregivers?

ҙ Is it possible for spirituality to flourish if the leadership does not support it? What about if the leadership is laissez-faire in regard to spirituality?

ҙ Reread Martha Loveland's suggestions. Are there additional suggestions you might make? If you were in leadership, which, if any, of her suggestions would you adopt? If you are in leadership, what do you do to make the workplace spiritually healthy?

Support for Spiritual Care

Overwhelmingly, the participants in this project believe that spiritual care is essential, and they each shared the ways they go about providing that care. Many also expressed frustration, however, about the lack of support for spiritual care. Much of this frustration is focused on the perception that today the margin is much more important than the mission in healthcare.

Pediatric nurse Carole Richards says, "I would like to see as much focus put on the patient as is put on money. I would like to see a greater commitment to meeting spiritual needs and a greater recognition that the nurse makes an important contribution to this care."

Dee Brooks explains that a stronger and more direct approach regarding spiritual care is needed: "From the beginning of the admission process we should ask patients what they desire for spiritual care. Then we need to follow up to make sure these needs are met and then we need to evaluate whether or not we were able to satisfy the spiritual needs of patients."

Dianne Smith agrees but observes that a stronger and more direct approach must be taken regarding expectations of competency for staff in providing spiritual care: "The focus on spirituality must be more than a brief mention during staff orientation. It must flow through every aspect of the healthcare experience." She believes that if spiritual care were truly valued, then financial support would be made available to staff for attending conferences and in-services as a way of increasing competence in this area. Dianne's suggestion is in line with a new standard mandated by the Joint Commission on the Accreditation of

Healthcare Organizations requiring a spiritual assessment on all patients admitted to a general hospital, all psychiatric patients, patients in long-term care, and patients receiving homecare services.[1]

A few respondents identified a need for greater support for spiritual interventions such as prayer and talking about a patient's relationship to God. Joyce Kinstlinger would like to see "a more open attitude for encouraging spirituality. This would include allowing staff to suggest to open and willing patients that bringing their problems to a Higher Power might be helpful. We should also be able to encourage patients to use churches, synagogues, and mosques as resources. And we should be allowed to encourage prayer in our patients' lives without fear of retribution."

Charity Johansson clarifies the difficult position that healthcare providers find themselves in when trying to balance agency policy with the responsibility to meet spiritual needs:

In the hospital, where I see patients once a week, as opposed to the educational setting, where I am the other days, I wish I would be given permission to spend some of my physical therapy minutes responding to a patient's spiritual needs. Right now I clock my minutes very specifically, for example, 2:04 to 3:03. Because I feel guilty spending any of these minutes on spiritual issues, I count any time spent responding to spiritual needs as nonbillable, nonproductive time. You know, not every patient wants a visit from the chaplain, and yet they may need some spiritual response every day. This part of care needs to be recognized as important.

"Respect for all persons is essential," adds Sandra Brown. "Patient-focused care needs to be supported in reality, not just in word. This support needs to include a thorough assessment of spiritual needs as well as provision of time and resources in the plan of care for meeting the spiritual needs of the patient. I believe that when a patient is in the hospital, it is essential that there be a designated spiritual leader who assesses the spiritual needs of patients every day and sees to it that those needs are met. This would include mobilizing the support systems that the patient values."

Occupational therapist Jay Brashear shares his dream for a spiritually centered home health agency: "I have a dream of starting my own home healthcare agency made up of clinicians and staff that are devoting their lives to the Lord. At our case conferences, we would pray for patients as well as discuss them. Somehow I would like this agency to challenge the current system nationally that makes accountability less documentation-driven. I would like to see the care of the patient take precedence over the care of the chart."

Nancy Shoemaker, who works in a clinic of a large private nonprofit hospital system, would like to see "a visible presence of interdenominational clergy, such as chaplains, making rounds in the patient and staff areas. I remember when I was hospitalized to deliver my children, I was in a Catholic hospital, and nuns stopped by every shift to say hello. I was very comforted by their presence. I believe that patients and staff alike would benefit from increased accessibility to people who have dedicated their lives to spiritual values."

Kay Hurd says that although she is greatly supported in her workplace, "I would like to see the chapel more accessible to patients, families, and staff. I also would like nursing education to instill a sense of 'caring for' patients and not just 'taking care of' patients. Many nurses are not taking care of the same patients every day, so that interconnectedness and relationships cannot be established. If one could work out a schedule so that nurses could care for the same patients, I believe it would help not only the nurse but the patient as well."

Patient-focused care needs to be supported in reality, not just in word. This support needs to include a thorough assessment of spiritual needs as well as provision of time and resources in the plan of care for meeting the spiritual needs of the patient. I believe that when a patient is in the hospital, it is essential that there be a designated spiritual leader who assesses the spiritual needs of patients every day and sees to it that those needs are met. This would include mobilizing the support systems that the patient values.

—Sandra Brown

REFLECTIONS

⌘ In what ways is spiritual care to patients and families supported in your workplace?

⌘ What would you like to see in your workplace to support the provision of spiritual care?

⌘ What are your thoughts about praying with patients? When, if ever, is this acceptable?

⌘ How do you give spiritual care to patients and families?

Support for Spiritual Care of Staff

Although all our participants identified the many ways that they nurture their own spirits, many of them also felt that the current healthcare system challenges their spirituality. Many of our respondents indicated that there is a need for a "culture" change regarding how people treat each other. Commenting on the importance of this, internist Herman Brecher contends, "There is nothing that needs to be done in the physical environment. What is crucial lies in the quality of the interpersonal relationship. It is in the interpersonal relationship that spirituality or belief is or is not created."

Family physician Bernita Taylor believes that improved communication at every level of healthcare would go a long way toward enhancing the spiritual climate. Carole Richards commented on the lack of mutual support that exists between co-workers and between supervisory staff and those who they supervise.

A common response among our respondents was the need for recognition of how important their work is. The current culture in healthcare with its focus on economic issues not only devalues patients but caregivers as well. Everything seems to be subordinate to the bottom line. Psychiatric nurse specialist Vicki Germer believes that healthcare workers need to hear more about the meaning of their work and a lot less about the financial concerns. Carol Story would like to be valued for the work that she does as a nurse, to be recognized and affirmed by those who are challenged to grow and succeed in their ministry as a result of her work.

A few respondents shared their frustration when their spiritual values and beliefs seem to be disregarded as unimportant. Harriet Coeling, on the nursing faculty of Kent State University, wishes that others would recognize her desire to put God first and to interpret things from God's perspective. She believes that her Christian faith tradition is not respected. Psychiatric nurse specialist Evelyn Yapp wants those in her work environment to show understanding rather than indifference to the importance of her spirituality: "I want them to look beyond the surface and recognize another person's internal qualities. I want them to make thoughtful decisions without greed in provision of healthcare to the people of God."

Several people identified the need for a quiet place to retreat to during the day. Nurse Elizabeth Page "would like to see a place set up so that people of all religions could go in and pray privately during the day." Vicki Germer commented that her facility had recently added a prayer-meditation room, and that it is a wonderful addition. Kelly Preston cited the need for "spiritual renewal days" that she believes could be sponsored by the chaplaincy department. Similarly, Charity Johansson adds, "There needs to be more openly sanctioned time for renewal of body and soul, less productivity expectations, and less committee time." Karen McCauley offers this observation regarding the impact of deadlines and productivity standards: "In homecare, everything is driven by deadlines and quotas. People tend to rush into the office from making visits in order to make the deadline and fail to take time to smell the roses. Less hectic schedules would go a long way to creating a spiritual environment."

From a parish nurse perspective, Catherine Lick adds:

I work in a church, but I feel that more could be done for and with the staff to create and foster relationships and support. This could be done through staff retreats that focus on personal care and concern, as well as on the real-

> **What is crucial lies in the quality of the interpersonal relationship. It is in the interpersonal relationship that spirituality or belief is or is not created.**
> **—Dr. Herman Brecher**

> **There needs to be more openly sanctioned time for renewal of body and soul, less productivity expectations, and less committee time.**
> **—Charity Johansson**

ization that ministry "burns" people out and we have to continually be filling our lamps. I came upon a quote from Mother Teresa that speaks what I am trying to say:

"Don't think that love, to be true, has to be extraordinary. What is necessary is to continue to love. How does a lamp burn if it is not by the continuous feeding of little drops of oil? When there is no oil, there is no light. . . . Dear Friends, what are our drops of oil in our lamps? They are the small things from every day life, the joy, the generosity, the little good things, the humility, and the patience, a simple thought for someone else. Our way to be silent, to listen, to forgive, to speak and to act, they are the real drops of oil that make our lamps burn vividly our whole life. Don't look for Jesus far away. He is not there. He is in you, take care of your lamp and you will see him."

This is what needs to be practiced in the workplace, whether a church, hospital, or factory.

There is research that supports many of the suggestions made by our respondents. Writing about Catholic institutions, Bazan and Dwyer call for healthcare organizations to address the spiritual needs of managers, physicians, nurses, and other employees who may be experiencing deep pain about the meaning and purpose of life.[2] The authors suggest prayer support and compassion as effective spiritual interventions but also propose that healthcare organizations can alter their structure and culture to provide environments that invite and support employees in addressing their spiritual issues. Organizations can develop specific programs to address the spiritual yearnings of employees. Such programs could include availability of private spiritual direction, formal mentoring, renewal days or retreats, and spirituality programs for professionals. They emphasize how important it is that spirituality be considered in every activity undertaken by the organization—including recruiting. Resources should be allocated for expanded spiritual services; quiet places for reflection, meditation, and related classes; traditional retreats; and qualified personnel to address spiritual needs.

Graber and Johnson advocate additional strategies for healthcare organizations desiring to integrate spirituality.[3] These include the use of focus groups to identify core or common values, ethics, and a philosophy of care. Any program sponsored by the healthcare organization must respect the views of nonreligious staff and patients and establish guidelines regarding the extent and nature of spiritual support for patients.

REFLECTIONS

ᐅᕁ What do you need in the workplace to support your own spiritual well-being?

ᐅᕁ Reread Catherine Lick's comments on pages 55–56. How do you keep your lamp filled?

ᐅᕁ What impact do the demands of your job have on your spirituality?

Positive Responses

Not everyone had suggestions for change in the workplace. Nurse Beatrice Rosen feels supported in her workplace. "Part of my spirit is to look at life and my job with optimism," she says. "My boss appreciates this, as there tends to be enough pessimism to go around. I also am aware that my immediate supervisors have a personal relationship with God—their compassion for others is evident, and that supports me in what I do and think."

Physician Jack Hasson observes, "Most times, in the heat of battle, we do not appreciate how fortunate we are to be in situations to help others on a daily and hourly basis. I see this when I bring others with me on rounds who are not in the healthcare arena. To a man or woman, they tell me how rewarded they felt to experience what we experience daily and take for granted. We should have ways to remind ourselves of this fact."

LOCATING THE IDEAL

We researched existing healthcare organizations to determine if there were any that embody what our participants are looking for. There are probably many, but we report on three models. We learned about the first one from one of the participants in this project, Eileen Altenhofer.

Eileen volunteers at Highline Community Hospital, the only Planetree facility in the state of Washington.[4] In 2001, Highline Community Hospital was named one of the nation's top fifteen "hospitals with a heart" in the American Association of Retired Persons' July/August *Modern Maturity* magazine. For the past nine years, Highline Community Hospital has been working to bring the Planetree philosophy to life within the healthcare system.

The Planetree Model

Planetree was founded in 1978 as a nonprofit organization with a mission to personalize, humanize, and demystify the healthcare experience for patients and families. The organization is dedicated to cultivating healing in a pleasant, caring environment and is focused on patient-centered rather than provider-centered care, recognizing that each patient is a unique individual with physical, emotional, and spiritual needs. Because of this uniqueness, patients have a voice in the care provided. They are encouraged to ask questions, to make suggestions, and to participate in their care.

The Planetree Alliance currently consists of forty-seven innovative hospitals and healthcare institutions located across the United States and in Canada. These organizations are dedicated to implementing Planetree programs and developing, with Planetree and other alliance members, new and increasingly effective programs.

The Planetree philosophy at Highline Community Hospital is evident in a variety of ways. For instance, patient education is viewed as critical to demystifying medical care. Patients have access to information about their medical condition and available treatments through the Planetree Health Library and Family Education program. Eileen Altenhofer volunteers at the library to do research for patients and families and to compile the research findings into a useful reference for them.

The patient-centered philosophy is expressed through the Healing Arts program, the environment, the respect and dignity afforded each patient and family, and the overriding belief that the patient is so much more than an illness. The patient is a whole person with emotional, physical, and spiritual needs who is member of a family, of a community, and of a culture.

Through the hospital's Healing Arts program, patients have access to chaplaincy services and the use of music, massage, warm-water therapy, relaxation techniques, aromatherapy, and other healing measures that result in greater comfort, less anxiety, and increased satisfaction for patients and families. The physical atmosphere of the facility is nurturing and as homelike as possible. The healing gardens at Highline offer a peaceful and beautiful sanctuary for patients, families, and staff.

In addition, Highline's patient care areas are designed to provide comfortable and homelike surroundings for patients and their guests. One of the wings of the hospital includes a spacious family area where families and friends can gather and relax and even make a meal in one of its full-size kitchens. Patients are cared for in private rooms with decorated woodwork, artwork, and large windows that foster a healing environment.

Medical-Religious Partnerships

A second model we found was developed by Daniel Hale and Richard Bennett in central Florida.[5] This model combines healthcare and spirituality in a different way than does Highline Community Hospital. Dr. Hale and Dr. Bennett have created partnerships between religious and healthcare organizations that build healthier communities. In contrast to the example of Highline Community Hospital, which incorporates the sacred into the secular healthcare arena, this project incorporates secular healthcare into the sacred arena of the church.

In these partnerships, the clergy speak from the pulpit to remind church members about the importance of maintaining health and seeking out quality healthcare for themselves and their families. When health is spoken about in the context of the church, health becomes more than a physical matter—it is a spiritual matter clearly linked to an individual's responsibility to honor the body as a temple of God's Spirit. Following the clergy's introduction of the importance of health as a relevant concern of the church, the congregation receives visits from doctors and other health professionals to provide education on important health issues such as cancer, hypertension, depression, and medication management. Additionally, the healthcare professionals provide training to church-based lay health educators and patient advocates. Hale and Bennett report that this model is so popular that it has spread beyond Christian congregations to Jewish synagogues and Muslim mosques.

Daughters of Charity Model

A third model, similar to Highline Hospital but with a religious foundation, is found in many of the hospitals that are part of the Daughters of Charity National Health System (DCNHS). In 1989, the leaders of the DCNHS-East Central region decided to explore the spirituality that was foundational to their ten facilities. They convened a study group made up of the top DCNHS-EC leaders and representatives of other DCNHS regions and ministries. They met quarterly for one year to explore the distinction between religion and spirituality, the difference between human development and human formation, the primacy in Western culture of the functional dimension of human life over the transcendent dimension, and the importance of beholding the mystery of life rather than trying to control or manipulate it.[6]

They completed their sessions in 1990 and summarized their findings. The leaders of each DCNHS-EC facility were encouraged to read, understand, and support the findings. The vice presidents for mission services were encouraged to integrate spirituality and spiritual formation in their work. Since that time, the DCNHS-EC facilities have integrated spirituality into the workplace by sponsoring spirituality committees, retreats, renewal days, and pilgrimages.

Let's take a look at one of those facilities, St. Vincent Hospitals and Health Services in Indianapolis, to see what it means when an institution integrates spirituality.

St. Vincent Hospitals and Health Services in Indianapolis is a tertiary hospital serving over 150,000 patients a year. The hospital is committed to treating the whole patient—body, mind, and spirit—and recognizes that healing cannot take place unless all aspects of the person are included in the care. The mission of the hospital extends beyond the walls of the institution to provide care for the poor and those whom the rest of society ignores. The hospital envisions itself as a catalyst for collaborative community action to provide a full range of preventive, social, spiritual, and educational services.

The hospital is the home of the Indiana Heart Institute, which is the state's largest cardiac center and one of the largest cardiac programs in the United States. In addition to the cardiac specialty, St. Vincent provides treatment for many other specialties such as cancer, sleep disorders, orthopedics and sports medicine, maternity care, neurology and neurosurgery, ophthalmology, hand and microsurgery, laser surgeries, minimally invasive surgeries, occupational health, stress centers, senior services, and community development. Additionally, an outreach service through St. Vincent Health provides healthcare to people who live in rural communities.

Part of St. Vincent's mission is to build better communities. The hospital offers a full range of community services. Let's examine just two areas where community contributions are made. In the area of the spiritual environment, St. Vincent's believes it is essential that the values, collaborations, and actions of individuals and communities reflect their beliefs and ethics, as well as a sense of being part of something bigger. They provide pastoral care counselors who strive to be conduits of God's love and peace for those who are confronted with life's struggles. Chaplains are available to provide comfort and guidance to patients and families while at the same time respecting individual faith preferences.

The hospital built the Seton Cove Spirituality Center as a place for spiritual growth. This interfaith center is available to St. Vincent staff for the purpose of spiritual formation and renewal. Spiritually focused programs are offered that provide insights into the spiritual significance of work and family life. In addition, St. Vincent physicians have received John Templeton Spirituality in Medicine grants in recognition of their efforts to integrate spirituality into resident programs and standards of care.

The hospital's commitment to the natural environment is evident in several ways. St. Vincent's Meditation and Fitness Trail is open to St. Vincent staff, patients, and the community at large. The trail provides a peaceful natural setting that fosters mental, physical, and spiritual well-being. The Reflection Garden is located in a quiet courtyard of the St. Vincent Hospital in Indianapolis and is dedicated to those in need of peace and spiritual strength to overcome the challenges of life. The Robert E. Colvin Simplicity Garden was donated by the family of a former St. Vincent staff member who provided the hospital with twenty-four years of loyal and dedicated service. The garden is surrounded by the walls of St. Vincent Hospital and includes a statue of St. Francis of Assisi to welcome visitors.

The hospital's commitment to education is evident in the Pediatric Asthma program, which provides a respiratory therapist to bring asthma education and therapies directly to school children suffering from asthma and other respiratory problems. St. Vincent's provides graduate, undergraduate, and continuing education opportunities to physicians, residents, and medical students with approved training in internal medicine, family medicine, obstetrics/gynecology, and geriatric medicine. Because St. Vincent recognizes that caring for the soul is essential to healing, it provides education and pastoral care residency programs in the Stress Center, hospice, cardiology, ICU, and family life areas. Other trained seminarians, clergy, and laypeople provide pastoral care in clinical areas throughout the hospital. St. Vincent has shared clinical pastoral education with hospitals in several adjacent communities. And lastly, St. Vincent collaborates with the University of Indianapolis and Marian College to sponsor registered nurses in a parish nurse course. This effort supports many denominations in the community in an effort to improve the health of all citizens. This is a healthcare system that has truly committed itself to the integration of spirituality in every aspect of its operations.

REFLECTIONS

- ⸎ Review the three models presented. In what ways do they integrate spirituality?
- ⸎ How does your workplace integrate spirituality?
- ⸎ What can you do to bring spirituality into the workplace?

THE VISION

Let's end this chapter with a bit of a fantasy excursion. We have heard about our participants' "wish list" regarding what they think would make the workplace more spiritual. We have examined three models that approximate elements of the ideal. Now, let's imagine the ideal. Allow the story of Pleasantville, a make-believe community, spark your imagination. Allow yourself to dream about what it would be like to work in Pleasantville Community Hospital or to provide healthcare service within the surrounding Pleasantville community.

Ten years ago the leadership in Pleasantville Community Hospital, desiring to differentiate itself from that of the other hospital systems in Pleasantville, conducted a large survey of the community. They were interested in knowing what factors influenced patients' choices regarding which healthcare facility and healthcare providers to use. The results of the survey indicated overwhelmingly (but not surprisingly) that respondents identified competence of healthcare providers as the most important factor in choosing a provider and/or a hospital. But in addition to provider competence, respondents identified other "soft factors" as almost equally important. The need to be treated with compassion and dignity, to be consulted on their care, and most of all to have their stories heard—all of these weighed heavily in respondents' healthcare choices. The hospital followed this large survey with focus groups to better understand what respondents wanted and how the hospital could ensure that these needs were met. The focus groups identified as spiritual issues these "soft factors" of patients being heard and feeling that they were not only receiving care but also being cared for.

The hospital administration followed the survey and focus groups with an investigative group charged with examining research literature in the area of patient satisfaction. These efforts led to the identification of a growing body of research pointing to the positive relationship between faith and health. The hospital decided to embark on a plan to systematically address spiritual issues as part of its mission to the Pleasantville community. The plan involved multiple steps, including:

1. Defining a new mission statement

2. Engaging all employees within the system to share the vision and to provide their input into implementation of the vision

3. Discovering what employees identify as essential supports for their own spiritual wholeness

4. Enlisting the support of hospital chaplains to plan a spiritual training program

5. Training existing employees as well as orienting new employees to this holistic approach

6. Modifying written materials used in all aspects of care, from admission to discharge, to reflect the holistic focus of the institution

7. Evaluating the environment to ensure that it supports spiritual well-being

8. Reaching out to the surrounding faith communities to collaborate on the development of congregational health ministries, including parish nurses and well-trained lay volunteers

9. Applying for a research grant to evaluate the effectiveness of these changes

10. Making a commitment that the Pleasantville Hospital and surrounding faith communities would be a center of excellence for spiritual research and holistic healthcare

11. Planning how these changes would affect day-to-day operations

Each of these steps is described.

The mission statement. The first step involved redefining the mission statement of the hospital. This process took six months to complete. The goal was to create a mission statement that was ecumenical in nature, that could capture the hearts and minds of the employees within the hospital system, and that would send a powerful message to the surrounding community that the hospital had indeed heard what people were asking for and was committed to providing not only competent healthcare but spiritual care as well. The following mission statement represents the culmination of these efforts:

We are a community of caregivers dedicated to service, respecting the religious and spiritual values of all who seek our services, bringing wholeness to patients and

families who come to us for care, facilitating wholeness in those who provide care, and making a difference through service to the community at large.

Involving staff in implementing the vision. Step two of the hospital's transformation involved engaging all employees within the Pleasantville Hospital system to share the vision and to seek their input into the implementation of the vision. This process took another six months and involved small-group discussions. The participants included chaplains, physicians, nurses, therapists, social workers, nursing assistants, and unit secretaries, as well as housekeeping, maintenance, admitting, billing, laboratory, dietary, and radiology employees—in fact, everyone who had any interpersonal contact with patients and families. The administration of the hospital assumed responsibility for sharing the results of the earlier investigative work. That research uncovered what patients wanted from the hospital, supporting the importance of integrating spiritual care into the total package of care and the importance of each employee in making this commitment to holistic care a reality. Out of these small-group discussions, the administration achieved "buy in" from the employees, who also provided suggestions regarding what was needed to support their own spiritual well-being.

Spiritual supports for staff. Step three involved discovering what employees believed were necessary spiritual supports for them. The suggestions made by employees included provision of places for quiet reflection, availability of ecumenical worship services throughout the day on all shifts, support of prayer groups, and spiritual retreats.

Development of training materials. Step four involved engaging the chaplains, the "spirituality experts," in developing training materials for existing employees as well as for new employees being oriented to the hospital system. The training included information about the importance of spiritual care; the relationship between religion and spirituality and how to respect each; how to recognize spiritual needs and implement spiritual care; how to fully integrate hospital chaplains and community-based clergy into the care delivery system; the importance of volunteerism; and what it means to be a good steward of limited resources.

Implementation of training. Step five commenced with the first training session provided to hospital personnel. Initially, chaplains used a "train the trainer" approach to provide instruction to personnel who were interested in becoming trainers. This approach decreased the burden on chaplains and greatly expanded the number of personnel with expertise in spiritual care. The training sessions were offered at a variety of times on all shifts to ensure that everyone was included. The training sessions were designed to be not just an exchange of information but rather a positive spiritual experience where participants shared their stories and learned from each other. The groups were small and always began with a prayer led by one of the participants. Refreshments were served, and participants left with a prepared booklet providing concrete examples of patient situations that exemplified spiritual care.

Revision of paperwork. The sixth step was tedious to complete. The administration recognized that creating a spiritual environment where wholeness could be achieved meant that every aspect of what the hospital did, including the forms and variety of paperwork used, needed to reflect this commitment. Beginning with the admission packet and moving though each piece of the record, every item of written material was scrutinized; much of it was changed. For instance, the following statement was added to letters sent to patients detailing what to expect during admission:

Pleasantville Hospital, in conjunction with a variety of faith communities, is dedicated to providing holistic care that includes meeting spiritual needs. Patients and families can expect that at least one person on the care team—a physician, nurse, chaplain, or social worker—will do a spiritual assessment/history and ask in what ways the patient can be supported spiritually during his/her hospital stay.

Structured assessment tools used by various healthcare providers were modified to include the spiritual aspect of care. Another critical decision was made to place plaques proclaiming the mission statement strategically throughout the hospital.

Environmental modification. Step seven involved an evaluation of the environment to determine whether it was conducive to spiritual well-being. This evaluation led to a decision to modify all areas of the hospital to be in line with the existing birthing center, where rooms were warm and inviting, and to designate "quiet reflection places" throughout the hospital where employees, patients, families, and other visitors could retreat for brief periods for spiritual recharging. Decisions were made to repaint all areas of the hospital in soothing colors and to play soft background music to create a peaceful ambience. The changes to the environment were phased in as part of a four-year capital improvement plan.

Inviting the community to participate. The eighth step ran concurrently with many of the earlier steps and focused on reaching out beyond the hospital boundaries to surrounding faith communities, business leaders, and other community-based health providers. This step was undertaken to expand the notion of a healing community from the hospital system to encompass the whole community. The Pleasantville Hospital system offered to fund a full-time position for a parish nurse coordinator. Faith communities were encouraged and offered support in developing congregational health ministries under the leadership of a parish nurse, who would be supported by the hospital-based parish nurse coordinator. Business leaders were encouraged to lend financial support to faith communities in their development of the parish nurse position as well as the congregational health ministry. Community-based healthcare providers were invited to participate actively in the unfolding of the hospital's vision, including attending the training sessions being offered.

Funding and research. The ninth and tenth steps were intricately linked. Pleasantville applied for and received a large research grant to evaluate the effectiveness of these system-wide changes. It sought the expertise of an internationally recognized medical researcher to provide leadership for the research efforts and made a commitment that the hospital, in conjunction with the surrounding community, would be a center of excellence in whole-person care.

Restructuring patient care. The eleventh step led to a major restructuring of how patient care was delivered. To provide the type of care to which the hospital had committed itself, additional resources were needed, and a new model of care was formulated. For instance, the essential role of the chaplain as the spiritual leader was recognized, but the hospital didn't have enough chaplains to provide the amount and type of support needed. Not only did the hospital undertake a major recruiting effort to hire more full-time chaplains, but it also made a commitment to establish Pleasantville Community Hospital as a chaplaincy training institution.

Another structural change involved inviting clergy from the surrounding community to provide religious services in the hospital chapel. These services were videotaped and could be accessed on closed-circuit television throughout the hospital. The chaplains interacted with patients, families, and all the staff who so desired.

A weekly care-planning meeting was added to each unit's schedule. This meeting included everyone who had contact with patients and families—physician, chaplain, nurses, social workers, therapists, nursing assistants, the parish nurse from the patient's faith community, and sometimes the housekeeping personnel. The focus of this meeting was to determine what the patients needed medically, emotionally, and spiritually, how those needs would be met, who on the team could best address specific needs, and what would be needed upon discharge to continue to move patients towards wholeness.

Usually any change is confronted with resistance; change is difficult and moves people out of their comfort zone. But at Pleasantville Community Hospital, where the changes were more than cosmetic and targeted the very culture of the hospital and surrounding community, change was embraced and applauded. The response of patients was so positive that there were waiting lists for admission for elective procedures. There was no nursing shortage at Pleasantville Community Hospital. In fact, nurses from all over the state applied for positions. The hospital served as a magnet for extraordinary practitioners in all fields who desired to work in an environment where the patient was the bottom line. Finances were not an issue either. The surge in patient revenue, together with donations from wealthy benefactors from the business community and a number or private foundations, supported the hospital's efforts.

Too good to be true? Perhaps, but maybe . . .

[4]

Preparation for Spiritual Caregiving

*Someday, after we have mastered the winds, the waves, the tides
and gravity, we shall harness for God the energies of love. Then
for the second time in the history of the world man will have
discovered fire.*

—Teilhard de Chardin

Let's begin this chapter with the experience of a nurse who "accidentally" became involved in providing spiritual care. Susan Feldman tells her story:

*My decision to become a nurse only surfaced after I started taking courses at our
local community college. I married within one year of graduating from high
school. When I was thirty-one years old, I experienced a strong desire to enroll
in my first college course. With the continued support of my husband and two
sons, one course followed another over the years. The challenge of the nursing curriculum always fascinated me and eventually led to a master's degree and to
Clinical Nurse Specialist certification in 1987 from the University of Maryland.
My original calling was based primarily on intellectual goals. I had a burning*

desire not only to achieve but also to excel. What happened genuinely surprised me.

I began my nursing career at Johns Hopkins Hospital. I quickly realized that what I had learned in the classroom paled in comparison to what I was learning through my clinical practice. The major change was in my own spirituality. It started with simple observations of the differences between patients and families with a strong belief in a higher power and those who did not espouse these beliefs. Many included me in their very personal prayers and thoughts. I was actually participating in a sacred trust between themselves and God. These impressions touched my life in ways that I cannot really explain. What I do know is that I slowly developed a profound sense of belonging, a connection to a higher being that ever since has touched my life daily.

I remember one experience when I was making nursing rounds on a Sunday morning and I opened the door to a patient's room. I found ten to twelve people surrounding the bed and praying together. I remember as I turned around to leave, they invited me to join them in prayer. It didn't matter that I was unfamiliar with their service. What mattered to them was that I was one more person who could deliver the power of prayer. It ended with their prayers over me—I left feeling very blessed.

Susan had no formal preparation to become a spiritual caregiver. One might recognize divine power moving in and through her to transform not only her nursing practice, but her heart as well, to provide spiritual care. It is love and compassion for others and the recognition, as Susan states, that we are part of a sacred trust between the patient and God. The question arises, however—should there be formal preparation for participation in this sacred trust, or should it be left to chance?

Our belief is that an essential aspect of making the healthcare system a spiritually healthy environment involves preparation of caregivers to understand the importance of the spirit, to recognize spiritual issues, and to be able to respond from the heart to these issues. Although an increasing number of medical and nursing schools incorporate spirituality courses into their curricula, many of these courses are electives. This means that the majority of students do not participate in any formal spiritual education process.

Another consideration is the large numbers of professionals who not only lack preparation in this area, but may have graduated and entered professional practice at a time when even discussing spiritual issues was discouraged by healthcare educators. Until this content is a requirement in the education of healthcare providers, it must be included in the orientation process of healthcare facilities to ensure that spiritual needs are addressed as part of holistic care.

As of 2003, the Joint Commission on the Accreditation of Healthcare Organizations (JCAHO) mandates that a spiritual assessment be completed on all patients admitted to a general hospital. There are four other groups who may receive treatment in specialty units/facilities for whom a spiritual assessment is also required: (1) terminally ill patients; (2) patients with a substance abuse diagnosis; (3) patients requiring pain management; and (4) psychiatric patients. In addition, the JCAHO Long Term Standards require that every patient in a long-term facility have a spiritual assessment completed and recorded in the chart.[1]

A structured approach assures the "head" knowledge while laying a foundation for the "heart" response that is the essence of spiritual care. It is essential that healthcare providers believe their role is to provide holistic care, and that means dealing not only with broken bodies, but broken minds, hearts, and souls.

REFLECTIONS

- Did you receive formal preparation regarding spiritual care? If so, what did that preparation entail?
- Do you believe that your preparation was adequate?
- Does your institution provide structured support in developing spiritual care expertise?
- Does your place of practice require a spiritual assessment?
- Reread Susan Feldman's story. What are your reactions to her statement that she was participating in a sacred trust between the patient and family and God?

What comprises the body of knowledge regarding spiritual care? What would a curriculum on spiritual care look like? We believe that the core content of such a curriculum includes topics such as:

- The differences between religion and spirituality
- The beliefs and practices of the world's major religions
- The influences of cultural beliefs and practices
- The intersection of legal and ethical issues with medical concerns and religious beliefs
- The ethical issues for the professional regarding appropriate boundary issues
- The importance and technique of conducting a spiritual assessment
- The appropriate spiritual interventions to respond to identified needs

The remainder of this chapter focuses on all these topics, except conducting a spiritual assessment and intervening to meet spiritual needs, which are discussed in chapter 5.

RELIGION AND SPIRITUALITY

In chapter 1, we differentiated spirituality from religion, concluding that spirituality refers to our relationship to God and our need to derive meaning and purpose from life events. There are additional dimensions of spirituality that need to be considered, however.

Belief and meaning refers to a person's beliefs that give meaning and purpose to life, major symbols that reflect meaning for this person, and the person's story.

Vocation and obligation refers to a person's sense of duty, obligation, or moral responsibility as a function of his or her beliefs.

Experience and emotion refers to experiences that a person has had in relation to the sacred, divine, or demonic, and what emotional significance these experiences hold for the individual.

Courage and growth refers to the ability to integrate the meaning of new experiences into existing beliefs and structures and/or the ability to let go of existing beliefs and symbols in order to allow new ones to emerge.

Community refers to participation in formal and informal communities where members share a common belief, meaning in life, and practices.

Authority and guidance refers to the source of authority for the person's beliefs and meaning in life, and in the person's vocation, practices, and rituals. Where does the person turn for guidance when faced with painful life situations? Does the person look within or without for guidance?

Transcendent values refers to values such as sanctity of life, the importance of truth telling, and the importance of treating others as we would like to be treated.

Spiritual qualities refers to personal qualities such as peace, joy, gratitude, forgiveness, forbearance, patience, and love.

Religion has a narrower focus than spirituality. Religion refers to our way of structuring and codifying our relationship with God. For many people, their religion provides the framework for the expression of their spirituality. The form of prayers and hymns, the manner in which formal religious services are conducted, the imposition of rules to guide moral and ethical behaviors, and the expectations for living one's life can all be found within a formal faith tradition and structure the ways that a person might approach God. However, this does not mean that religion and religious practice encompass all of spirituality. Dimensions of religiosity include:

- Chosen religious belief system
- Active participation within that faith community
- Adherence to specific religious observances
- Embracing principles and values of a specific faith tradition

Spirituality is much broader than religion and is inclusive, whereas religion tends to be exclusive, producing a sense of "us" and "them," "insiders" and "outsiders." Spirituality is relational, with the core of spirituality centered on a relationship with God. The significance of this core relationship, however, reverberates through and shapes all other important relationships. How we connect with family, friends, our communities, and our workplace, and even how we relate to ourselves are affected by our relationship to God. Art, music, crafts, cooking, woodwork, gardening, volunteer activities, and sports can all be influenced by the way a person views God's role in his or her life.

Spirituality is relational even in its focus on meaning and purpose. When people ask questions such as "Why me?" "Why now?" "What does it mean?" and "What difference do I make?" they are attempting to define the relationship of their lives to ultimate truth and reality. Our patients who struggle for answers as they attempt to deal with illnesses that ravage bodies, minds, and souls pose these questions. Healthcare providers who grapple with a healthcare system in spiritual crisis ask these same questions. These are ultimately spiritual issues, and they are deeply embedded not only in the stories of our patients but in our own stories as well.

> Spirituality is relational even in its focus on meaning and purpose. When people ask questions such as "Why me?" "Why now?" "What does it mean?" and "What difference do I make?" they are attempting to define the relationship of their lives to ultimate truth and reality.

We need to be aware that not all patients requiring our care are religious; they may not belong to a faith tradition; they may not attend regular worship services; and yet they may be deeply spiritual. Does this mean that we should not be concerned about religion? Absolutely not! In fact, most of the research that exists in this field examines the overwhelmingly positive relationship between religious practices such as praying and attending religious services and various health outcomes such as lowered blood pressure, less depression and anxiety, improved coping, shorter hospital stays, ability to resist alcohol and drug use, less death anxiety, increase in positive health behaviors, and use of preventive health services.[2]

Understanding the importance of religion is essential, because for many people their spirituality is expressed through the structure of their faith tradition. Our focus must be inclusive enough, however, that we recognize and respond to the spiritual needs of those who are not religious as well as those who are. Physician Daniel Ober suggests that respect is the key: "It is more than simply tolerance. Spirituality is often more than religious behavior—it is the very core of one's day to day activities."

Although it is not necessary that healthcare professionals be expert on all religions, it is important that they be open to the religious beliefs and spirituality expressed by patients and families. Physician Jack Hasson supports the need for structured preparation in this area: "An educational approach to beliefs and practices of others allows us to be more sensitive to these issues. We do not want to stress patients or employees further by doing or saying things that are contrary to their belief systems."

Family practitioner Bernita Taylor recounts an example of lack of respect for a physician's religious beliefs: "At one clinic where I worked, the administration did not want to allow a Muslim physician to leave every Friday to attend the prayers at the mosque. I volunteered to cover for him on a regular basis, as I felt it was discriminating to try to control his religious expression in this way. His beliefs were being belittled because he was a non-Christian."

> A structured spirituality curriculum not only assures the "head" knowledge but also lays a foundation for the "heart" response that is the essence of spiritual care. It is essential that healthcare providers believe their role is to provide holistic care, and that means dealing not only with broken bodies, but broken minds, hearts, and souls.

Martha Loveland, speaking from the perspective of a healthcare administrator, offers this perspective: "I think that management could benefit from sensitivity training done about various major national and international religions and denominations. In addition, I think management training could include data about demographic changes in church-affiliated membership, spiritual traditions, worship services. This information would be valuable to supervisors in helping them avoid awkward situations such as Jehovah Witnesse's not recognizing birthdays and Christmas." (See Appendix A for summaries of the beliefs and practices of major world religions.)

We asked participants how it is possible to simultaneously respect and encourage spirituality as well as respect religious differences. "It sometimes feels very tricky," says Vicki Germer, "but I just try to connect with the commonalties that we all share, such as a desire for love, meaning, and transcendence." Nurse Dianne Smith says, "The key is to maintain respect. There have been times when I have disagreed with the religious beliefs of others, and I have chosen either not to respond or to acknowledge that I disagreed with but respected their different beliefs. I believe that by showing others respect when they express their beliefs, I am encouraging freedom of expression."

We also asked for examples of how beliefs were respected within the healthcare environment. Marilyn Bullock, a nurse in a long-term-care facility, recalls taking care of an elderly gentleman whose Islamic beliefs dictated a small but significant change in nursing care: "We noticed that throughout the day, he would orient his wheelchair in a certain direction in the room. If we spoke to him at these times, he became disturbed with the staff. Finally we asked him what the problem was, and he told us that during these times he oriented his wheelchair towards the east and was engaged in praying. Once we became aware of the meaning of his behavior, we were respectful of his prayer times, and we reoriented his bed so that it faced the east—recognizing his need to pray toward Mecca."

CULTURAL INFLUENCES AND SPIRITUALITY

Culture plays a significant role in the expression of spirituality, and in turn both play a significant role in healthcare. For instance, cultural beliefs may include spiritual explanations for the causes and treatment of illnesses. Some cultures believe that the human soul can be lost, dislodged, or captured as a result of a traumatic experience or witchcraft. Many non-Western cultures revere the spiritual nature of plants, animals, mountains, water, and other nonhuman forms and believe that disrespect and disconnection from them can lead to illness. Other cultures look to supernatural spiritual forces such as ancestors and gods that may be kind, evil, or changing. In cultures that hold to these supernatural beliefs, people are expected to give offerings to these supernatural spirits, to act in ways that appease these spirits, or to protect the soul from capture through rituals or wearing amulets.[3]

Cultural factors also affect the perceived need for health services. For instance, Italians and Jewish people more readily recognize and express somatic concerns than those of Irish and English descent, who tend to minimize and deny symptoms. Culture may also affect how readily people seek out medical services.[4]

Lannin and colleagues explored the reasons that the mortality rate for breast cancer among African American women is higher than for white women. Among their findings was that cultural beliefs play a significant role in the stage at which breast cancer is diagnosed in African American women. Common to the women in this study were fundamentalist religious beliefs such as, "The devil can cause a person to get cancer" and "If a person prays about cancer, God will heal it without medical treatments." The researchers concluded that socioeconomic and cultural/spiritual beliefs accounted for the delay in diagnosis among African American women.[5]

Other cultures may view illness as a punishment from God; still others may take a fatalistic approach to illness—"If I am going to get sick, then there is nothing I can do about it." Such cultural/spiritual beliefs have an impact on healthcare. It is difficult to promote preventive care when the current of cultural belief runs counter to a sense of personal control.

REFLECTIONS

- Think about your experiences dealing with cultural beliefs different from your own. What were those beliefs? What was the most challenging aspect of dealing with these differences? How did you deal with these differences?
- How do you assess for cultural issues that may have a bearing on the delivery of healthcare?
- How does your personal cultural heritage affect your spirituality?

SPIRITUALITY, RELIGION, HEALTHCARE, AND THE LAW

There are healthcare situations—such as the need for immuniza-tions, blood transfusions, and medical treatments—that require patients and/or families to make decisions that may be counter to their religious beliefs. Likewise, healthcare providers may be faced with situations and decisions that also challenge their religious beliefs. These decisions rep-resent spiritual dilemmas for the patient and/or family, as well as for the healthcare providers involved in the care.

When faced with a healthcare choice that violates a religious tenet, people experience spiritual distress. Conversely, for the healthcare pro-fessionals involved in the care, the conflict centers on the desire to respect the patient's right to choose, while at the same time providing optimum care, and, in some instances, preserving life. In addition, the patient's choice may cause the healthcare professional to experience conflict with personal religious beliefs. This interface of healthcare treat-ment conflicting with religious belief and the role of the law is an area about which healthcare professionals require knowledge to be able to respond appropriately to patients and families and to be able to resolve their personal conflicts.

Under the "free exercise" establishment clause of the First Amend-ment to the U.S. Constitution, Congress is prohibited from making any law "respecting an establishment of religion." The Fourteenth Amend-ment extends this constitutional protection by prohibiting state govern-ments from intruding on certain religious freedoms.[6] The Tenth Amend-ment, however, allows state governments some leeway to protect the health and welfare of citizens. The degree to which the federal or state government may intrude on the exercise of religious beliefs is largely shaped by Supreme Court, federal court, and state court decisions.

Let's take a look at some situations where this conflict occurs.

Immunizations

Pediatricians, as well as community and school health nurses, are usually the professionals confronted with questions about immunizations. In late summer and early fall, as families prepare to send children off to school, parents are required to make sure their children receive state-mandated immunizations. Parents turn to healthcare professionals to learn which immunizations are required. They may also turn to these same healthcare professionals to express their concerns that these immunizations are a violation of their religious beliefs.

This puts the healthcare professional in a very difficult position. On one hand, state law mandates immunizations as a precondition for school enrollment. On the other hand, there is the family's sincerely held religious belief that immunizations should not be given to their child. The healthcare professional wonders if the state law regarding immunizations violates the family's free exercise of religion, but also whether the parents' decision is the best one for the child.

This issue seemed to have been settled in favor of the state's right to mandate vaccination as a precondition to public school attendance when the Supreme Court in 1905 ruled in *Jacobson v. Massachusetts* that the state's mandatory smallpox vaccination was constitutional. This decision was based on the conclusion that the state interest in protecting health was sufficiently strong to outweigh any religious beliefs that might be violated.[7]

A secondary issue, however, soon arose. A number of states began to provide exemptions for mandatory immunizations. To qualify for this exemption, people could either swear that they were members of an organized religion that opposed such immunizations, or they could produce a certificate from their church stating that the church opposed immunizations. These exemptions were challenged on the grounds that they unconstitutionally favored those belonging to an established religion over individuals who sought exemption but were not members of an organized church eligible for exemption.

Because the "establishment" clause of the First Amendment requires that all religious beliefs be treated equally, most state courts have found these "organized religion" exemptions to be unconstitutional.[8] If a state wants to allow an individual to refuse immunizations because of religious conviction, it must allow the refusal even if the person is not a member of an organized religion. This issue continues to be challenged by families claiming that their personal religious belief is sufficient to qualify for the religious exemption from immunizations.[9]

For nurses and physicians who are confronted with this situation, it is mandatory that they know exactly what immunizations are required and whether the state provides a religious exemption for mandatory vaccination. Fortunately, the issue of whether to vaccinate is not a crisis situation. However this could dramatically change if there were a biological attack by terrorists with a disease such as smallpox. Such a situation would require providers to immediately consider the religious implications of forced inoculations.

In cases where an adult or child requires a blood transfusion or surgical intervention, there may be little time for lengthy consideration of the patient's beliefs versus the value of the treatment protocol.

Blood Transfusions

Any healthcare professional who practices in a hospital setting is confronted with the need for patients to receive either a blood transfusion or blood products. Occasionally, a patient or patient's parents decline blood transfusions because of their religious tenets. Those who take this stand are usually members of the Jehovah's Witnesses. In some instances, the religious beliefs of the individual are honored, and the transfusion is withheld. In other instances, the transfusion is ordered against the wishes of the patient or parents. Sometimes these decisions seem irrational to the healthcare providers involved in the case and many times create confusion, distress, and anger among staff members.[10] Let's examine some relevant court decisions that shed some light on the logic behind these decisions.

Refusal by Jehovah's Witnesses to consent to blood transfusions has resulted in a great deal of litigation. The process usually begins with the hospital petitioning the local court for guardianship over the adult or custody of the child in order to obtain transfusion permission. The willingness of the court to grant custody to the hospital is to some degree based on whether the transfusion is needed to correct a life-threatening condition and whether the patient is an adult or a child.

Courts have examined a number of factors in deciding whether to compel an adult to receive a blood transfusion. For example, in the

Georgetown[11] case, the Circuit Court of the District of Columbia ordered a woman to receive a blood transfusion in connection with a bleeding ulcer. The court ordered the transfusion because the patient did not seem rational enough to make the decision, and she had a seven-month-old baby whom the community might have had to care for in the event of her death. In addition, the court found that the hospital and staff might be exposed to a lawsuit if the transfusion were withheld.

When faced with a healthcare choice that violates a religious tenet, people experience spiritual distress. Conversely, for the healthcare professionals involved in the care, the conflict centers on the desire to respect the patient's right to choose, while at the same time providing optimum care and, in some instances, preserving life.

Since *Georgetown*, several courts have analyzed surrounding circumstances and upheld transfusions against a patient's religious beliefs. An example in which the court honored the patient's religious wishes is the *Brooks* case.[12] Bernice Brooks suffered from a peptic ulcer. Mrs. Brooks, her husband, and her two adult children were all Jehovah's Witnesses. The patient and her husband agreed to sign a form releasing the physician and the hospital from civil liability for failure to administer a blood transfusion. Despite this, the hospital still desired to administer the transfusion. The Supreme Court of Illinois decided that the transfusion should not be ordered because Mrs. Brooks appeared competent to make the decision and there was no "clear and present danger" to society as a result of her decision.

In reviewing whether adults should receive compulsory blood transfusions, the courts have looked at such factors as whether the patient is mentally competent to refuse treatments, whether minor children will be affected by the patient's death, the duty the state owes to protect the public's interest in life, and the potential liability of the hospital and staff. The court's mandate attempts to balance these factors.

In the case of children, in life-threatening emergency situations, courts are likely to order blood transfusions even though they are contrary to parental religious beliefs. Conversely, in nonemergency situations, courts have been reluctant to act against parental religious beliefs to order transfusions.

Regardless of how a court rules in these cases, the patient and family are pitted against the very people who are committed to promoting health and preserving life. In terms of the spiritual consequences of these conflicts, no matter what the outcome, someone—either patient, family, or healthcare provider—loses.

Medical Treatments

There are two issues in regard to medical treatment that relate to spirituality. The first involves the rights of parents to choose faith healing over traditional medical treatment for their children. The second focuses on situations in which a healthcare provider might refuse to provide a treatment based on personal religious beliefs.

Faith healing versus medical treatment. Courts have generally interpreted the concept of freedom of religion very broadly to include both religious belief and religious practice, including the right to choose prayer and/or religious ritual in place of medical treatment for a disease or disorder.[13] When faced with a medical problem, an adult can seek medical attention, use faith healing, try alternative medical treatment, or pursue no treatment at all and let nature take its course. When parents or guardians wish to exercise the same options for their children, however, there is frequently serious conflict with healthcare professionals as well as civil authorities.

In 1974, the U.S. Department of Health, Education, and Welfare first required states to have clauses in their child abuse and neglect legislation that permitted exemptions on religious grounds. If a state refused to include these exemptions, it was prohibited from receiving federal child-abuse protection grants. By 1999, forty states had complied with the federal mandate. Parents who choose prayer in place of medical care for a sick or injured child cannot be prosecuted in states that recognize this religious freedom.

Although this federal regulation no longer exists, in 2002 thirty-eight states still had laws that permitted parents to reject medical treatment for their children in favor of faith healing.[14] The Academy of American Pediatrics, the American Medical Association, and the National District Attorneys Association have gone on record in opposition to these laws. Dr. Seth Asser, co-author of an article on medically preventable child fatalities, commented, "You can't beat, sexually abuse or starve your kids, but the law allows a parent to refuse medical treatment in favor of magic. This is not just a social phenomenon, but a public-health issue."[15]

One example of court involvement occurred in 1993, when Douglas Lundman sued his ex-wife and various Christian Science groups over the death of his eleven-year-old son in 1989. The boy had juvenile diabetes, and while under his mother's care, he had fallen into a diabetic coma and died. The jury found that the mother, Kathleen McKown, her new husband, the Christian Science practitioner, the Christian Science nursing home that provided his nurse, the local representative of the Christian Science publication, and the church itself shared responsibility for the boy's death. Mr. Lundman was awarded compensatory damages of over $5 million, and the church was assessed an additional $9 million in punitive damages. The compensatory damages were lowered to $1.5 million on appeal, but the church's punitive damages were not lowered. The case was appealed to the U.S. Supreme Court, which refused to review the case, thus letting the judgment stand.[16]

Right of a healthcare provider to choose. In 1999 a young woman, Guadalupe Benitez, a lesbian, was seeking to become pregnant by artificial means. Ms. Benitez was referred to North Coast Women's Care Medical Group in San Diego, California, where she underwent nearly a year's worth of infertility treatment. When this did not result in pregnancy, Ms. Benitez sought artificial insemination. Reportedly Dr. Christine Brody, a Christian, refused to perform the procedure on the grounds that artificially inseminating a homosexual violated the doctor's faith tradition. Dr. Brody referred Ms. Benitez to an outside physician who would complete the procedure.

Displeased by this action, Ms. Benitez sued Dr. Brody and the North Coast Women's Care Medical Group based on a California law that prohibits discrimination by healthcare providers and business organizations. A San Diego trial court found the case without merit and dismissed the lawsuit in 1999. However, Ms. Benitez appealed that decision, claiming that she was emotionally traumatized when she was unlawfully "dumped" as a patient due to her homosexuality.

She is supported by the Lambda Legal Defense, a group that works to gain rights for homosexuals. The group has asked the California Court of Appeals in San Diego to overturn the lower court decision and to compensate Ms. Benitez for a procedure that she claims should have been provided by her healthcare plan and the North Coast Women's Medical Clinic. Lambda Legal's position is that physicians are entitled to hold any personal religious beliefs they choose, but they do not have the right to refuse medically appropriate treatment to a patient based on what the physician claims are personal beliefs about particular groups of people.

If Lambda Legal succeeds in getting the lower court's ruling overturned, the consequences would be a serious assault on the right of physicians as well as other healthcare professionals to make decisions based on conscience. For instance, Christian physicians and nurses would be compelled to provide abortion counseling to young girls and to participate in abortions.[17] Agudath Israel of America, a Jewish lobbying group, expresses similar concerns that Jewish healthcare providers deserve legislative protection and should not be compelled to participate in medical procedures they find religiously or morally objectionable. Similarly, Agudath Israel argues that healthcare providers should not be compelled to discontinue medical treatment or to withhold nutrition or hydration if it would violate their beliefs to do so.[18]

REFLECTIONS

- As a healthcare provider, how can you institute measures to protect a patient's religious beliefs when those beliefs stand in opposition to accepted treatment modalities?
- Under what circumstances do you think that parents should be allowed to discontinue or withhold medical treatment for their child? In a situation where a parent made such a decision, in what ways do you think your own spiritual well-being would be affected?
- If a patient under your care died because he or she had refused treatment, what effect would this have on your spirit? How would you deal with this situation?

SPIRITUALITY, HEALTHCARE, AND
ETHICAL CONCERNS

Spirituality and religious beliefs, doctrine, and practice profoundly shape people's ethical behavior and their beliefs about life, sickness, and death. According to multiple surveys, the majority of Americans believe in the power of God or prayer to improve the course of an illness. As healthcare professionals, we must be sensitive to the power of these beliefs to influence views and decisions regarding issues such as end-of-life care, suicide, stem cell research, euthanasia, rationing of healthcare, and abortion.

Although Jewish and Christian beliefs dominate bioethical dialogue within the United States, we must be aware that these perspectives do not exhaust the possible perspectives on life, death, and medical intervention. We must be open to hearing the ethical concerns of Muslims, Hindus, Buddhists, and others from non-Western traditions.[19] Darryl Macer argues in "Bioethics Is Love of Life: An Alternative Textbook" that "most people find religion to be a much more important source of guidance in life than science. Any theory of bioethics that will be applied to peoples of the world must be acceptable to the common trends of major religious thought."[20]

> Although Jewish and Christian beliefs dominate bioethical dialogue in the United States, we must be aware that these perspectives do not exhaust the possible perspectives on life, death, and medical intervention. We must be open to hearing the ethical concerns of Muslims, Hindus, Buddhists, and others from different traditions.

In addition to the major bioethical issues mentioned above, it is essential that we consider the ethical concerns surrounding the provision of spiritual care. As healthcare providers, we are confronted with people of deep faith, people of questioning faith, and people of no faith. Regardless of where patients and families are on their own faith journeys, we must never impose our beliefs or practices on them.

Healthcare providers are in positions of power relative to our patients: we understand the mysterious workings of the body and mind; we use words that are incomprehensible to the patient; and we may engage in actions that violate the patient's personal boundaries. Great care must be taken to avoid using that power for spiritual manipulation. A patient should never feel coerced to believe or practice as we do. There should never be any suggestion that healthcare depends on the patient's or family's acceptance of our beliefs and/or practices. Likewise, we must avoid placing spiritual expectations on patients, implying that their recovery or lack of recovery is a result of the quality or degree of their faith.

Any such behavior on our part is disrespectful of the patient's spirituality and/or religious beliefs or lack thereof. This is spiritual abuse and has no place in the ministry of healthcare.

REFLECTIONS

- How has your faith shaped your position on various bioethical issues?
- Have you ever faced a situation that caused you ethical conflict? What was the situation? How did you resolve it? How did your spirituality and/or faith tradition influence the resolution?
- Have you ever worked with a patient or family that faced an ethical dilemma—perhaps it was over an end-of-life decision such as termination of treatment; perhaps it was about telling a patient a "truth" that was painful and would have serious consequences—and, if so, what was your role in supporting the patient or family in reaching a decision? What role did spirituality (the patient's, the family's, and your own) play in the decision?
- This chapter focused on aspects of the preparation to be a spiritual caregiver. In the next chapter, we examine ways to inquire about spiritual and religious beliefs and to provide spiritual interventions that are ethical, loving, and respectful of that sacred trust between our patients and God in which we are allowed to participate.

[5]

Providing Spiritual Care

Healing is not for you. . . . Without your wound where would
your power be? It is your very remorse that makes your low
voice tremble into the hearts of men. The very angels themselves
cannot persuade the wretched and blundering children on earth
as can one human being broken on the wheels of living. In
Love's service only the wounded soldiers can serve. Draw back.
—Thornton Wilder, *The Angel That Troubled the Waters*

This chapter deals with two topics: assessing spiritual needs and responding to those needs. Before we proceed with that discussion, the introductory quotation requires some explanation. It is taken from Thornton Wilder's play *The Angel That Troubled the Waters*, and it acknowledges a deep reality known by everyone who cares for the health needs of others—there is a reciprocal relationship between the sufferer and the healer. We share in the suffering of those for whom we provide ministry and comfort.

The play is based on the biblical story of the healing pool at Bethesda (John 5:2–9), but in Wilder's version, a physician seeks healing for himself at the pool. The physician is rebuffed by one of the invalids who spends her days at the pool waiting for the angel's touch to transform the waters into healing balm. The invalid tells the doctor that the pool is no place for a healer, especially one who appears so healthy. The angel, visible only to the physician, then appears and speaks the words in the introductory quotation. The invalid receives healing from the pool, but the physician is sent away to ponder the angel's message that only the wounded soldier is able to minister in Love's service.

Our primary task is one of love, albeit love matched with professional knowledge and skill, and our abilities to hear the stories of others and to respond to the deepest needs expressed in the stories frequently involves our own suffering.[1]

How do we know a person's spiritual needs? How do we know their spiritual history? How do we assess spirituality? Once we enter the spiritual dimension and begin to walk alongside the person we are serving, what do we do with the knowledge that we obtain? What do we do with the pain? Are there interventions that we can offer to bring comfort and peace, support hope, build connections, facilitate forgiveness and reconciliation, ease the pain of grief, respond lovingly to anger and rejection, and accompany others to the next chapter of their story? Even to begin to address these needs is a tall order for any healthcare professional, but the possibility exists, and in embracing the possibility we open ourselves to an expanded vision of caring—to the ministry of healthcare.

HEARING THE STORY

Learning about spiritual needs is referred to as "taking a spiritual history" in medicine and "assessing spiritual needs" in nursing. Although the language is slightly different, both approaches strive to understand the story of the patient.

This story—unlike the information obtained in a traditional history and physical, where we focus on past health issues, the current complaint, the history of various treatments, and the patient's response to those treatments, as well as the family and social history—reveals more than factual information. We are searching for the threads that weave the facts together and make them come alive. We are searching for the pattern in the person's life tapestry that allows us to see the fractured person in front of us as unique and precious with a story like no other.

Once we hear the story, there is no way this person who seeks our ministry can ever be just another "diabetic," or "dysfunctional neurotic," or "heart patient." Instead, we are able to glimpse what God sees when God looks at us, a creation that is wonderful and of inestimable value.

Many believe that inquiring about a person's story, asking about faith and religion and meaning, is itself an incredibly powerful intervention. We agree that this is so. The mere inquiry delivers a powerful message to the patient and family that we are truly interested in them—their wholeness, their brokenness, and their woundedness. And more than just being interested, for a period of time we are ready to accompany them on their journey; and even if it is painful, we are committed to the trip.

Before examining specific approaches for gathering spiritual information, let's examine the need to do a spiritual self-assessment.

SPIRITUAL SELF-ASSESSMENT

Before you begin to assess another's spiritual needs, it is important to take a look at yourself. What do you believe? How do you perceive God working in your own life? What do you think about the value of prayer? Where does your support come from? Shelly has compiled a list of spiritual self-assessment questions, which we reproduce here for your review.[2] As you read through them, consider either entering into a dialogue with another person and sharing your answers with that person, or writing your answers in a journal so you can reread and reflect on them.

What do you remember about your childhood? How would you describe family relationships then and now?

What other significant relationships do you have? How did they develop? What are these relationships like? Describe them.

If you are a parent, describe your relationship with your child(ren). Are there other children in your life with whom you relate? Describe those relationships.

What events in your life stand out as the most significant? Why?

When did you first learn about God? How was God presented to you?

How did you experience God's presence as a child?

What is your image of God?

As you reflect on your life, are there crisis points in your relationship to God? What circumstances surrounded the crisis? How did your relationship to God change?

What person(s) played the most significant role in your faith development?

How have the most significant relationships of your life (spouse, parent, best friend, etc.) influenced your faith journey?

What is your faith community like? What influence does this community have on your faith journey?

What rituals, disciplines, or religious practices have been helpful or meaningful to you?

Where do you receive spiritual support?

What kind of spiritual support do you need? Are you receiving it?

Describe a time when you were angry with God. How did you work through this period?

How do you experience God working through your life right now?

In what way does your faith help you in your daily life?

How has your faith influenced the major decisions in your life?

How has your relationship to God influenced your care for others?

What spiritual resources do you draw upon when you feel overwhelmed?

REFLECTIONS

- Reread the opening quotation from Thornton Wilder's play. How do you deal with the pain of ministry? Where does your healing come from?

- How do you initiate "hearing the patient's story"?

- Are there times when you consciously choose to "not hear the story"? What circumstances would influence such a decision?

ᴈ⋆ What are the differences in your healthcare ministry between when
you open yourself up to the patient's story and when you don't?

ᴈ⋆ What difference do you think it makes to your healthcare ministry
that you are spiritually self-aware?

MEDICINE'S APPROACH

Those unfamiliar with spiritual assessment raise questions about how
to approach the area of spirituality, the timing of the inquiry, which
patients are candidates for a spiritual history, and what should be asked.
Frequently the patient opens the door to spiritual inquiry by directly
mentioning his religious faith.[3] A comment such as "I have been praying that God will heal me" is an open invitation to the healthcare
provider to explore this area. This opening seems to give the healthcare
provider tacit approval for further inquiry regarding spiritual and religious issues.

It is not sufficient, however, to wait for the patient to provide this
opportunity. The spiritual history should be a structured part of the
physician's initial conversation with a patient. King[4] suggests that taking
a spiritual history should be part of the social history obtained by the
doctor as part of all outpatient physical examinations, as well as for all
patients admitted to the hospital. This is a responsibility that the physician should not delegate, even if nursing, social work, and the chaplaincy service are also inquiring about spiritual issues. Doctors need to
know about any factor that has as powerful an effect on the patient's
medical decision-making as their religious or spiritual beliefs.[5]

Although several studies report that many patients also support the
need for the physician to conduct a structured spiritual history, the reality is that very few patients ever experience this.[6] It is important that the
physician be sensitive to the possibility that the patient and family may
seem surprised and even a bit uncomfortable when the topic of spirituality is first introduced. This can be handled by an introductory comment by the physician such as, "I want to ask you a few questions about
your spiritual and religious beliefs. This may seem like an unusual topic
for us to discuss, but research shows that for many patients this area is

significant to their healing. Since I am interested in your well-being, I am interested in whatever supports you in maintaining health and getting better."

The importance of a spiritual assessment increases for the hospitalized patient, and serious medical issues magnify the significance of spiritual concerns. This is especially true for patients who are admitted to intensive care, are terminally ill, are facing surgery, are suffering from a severe psychiatric illness, or are receiving long-term care. As mentioned in chapter 4, JCAHO mandates a spiritual assessment for these categories of patients. Patients who are confronting serious medical issues—such as whether to choose active treatment versus palliative care—are many times influenced more by their values regarding the sanctity of life and their religious beliefs than they are by medical explanations and prognostic predictions. This is supported by a study of 177 consecutive patients seen in the pulmonary clinic at the Hospital of the University of Pennsylvania. Nearly half of all patients (45 percent) indicated that if they became gravely ill, religious beliefs would influence their medical decisions.[7]

Similarly, a survey of 100 patients with advanced lung cancer, their families, as well as 257 medical oncologists attending the annual meeting of the American Society of Clinical Oncology, asked them to rank the importance of the following seven factors that might influence chemotherapy treatment decisions: oncologist's recommendation, faith in God, ability of treatment to cure the disease, side effects of the treatment, family doctor's recommendation, spouse's recommendation, and children's recommendation.[8] The patients and their families and physicians ranked the recommendation of the patient's oncologist first. Although patients and family members both ranked faith in God second, however, oncologists ranked faith in God last (seventh). This study demonstrates that health professionals often underestimate the role that religious beliefs play in coping and the influence they have on decisions that affect the patient's care.

Religious beliefs influence many healthcare decisions made by patients. Adherence to a diet; compliance with medical treatment, including medications; acceptance of blood products; vaccination of children; participation in prenatal care; follow-through, with referrals to either a psychiatrist or a psychologist; and end-of-life decisions may all be profoundly influenced by a patient's and family's religious beliefs. A physician who is knowledgeable about the spiritual beliefs and religious practices that will ultimately affect these decisions is better prepared to help patients and families through their struggle.[9]

What constitutes a spiritual history, and how is such a history taken? In general terms, the spiritual history attempts to gather information about the patient's belief in God, religious beliefs and practices, and sense of purpose and meaning, as well as how these beliefs influence the patient's ability to cope with illness and decisions about medical care. In collecting this information, we are identifying spiritual needs, including (1) the need to love and be loved in return, (2) the need to experience and extend forgiveness to others, and (3) the need to find meaning and purpose in life and hope for the future.[10]

Although there are a number of instruments available to take a spiritual history, it is not essential that the physician use one of these instruments. We believe it is more important to conduct the spiritual history in a sensitive and respectful manner and to collect complete information.[11] The following are the essential areas to include:

• Does the patient use religion or spirituality to help cope with illness, or is religion a source of stress, and how?

• Is the patient a member of a supportive spiritual community?

• Does the patient have any troubling spiritual questions or concerns?

• Does the patient have any spiritual beliefs that might create conflicts with his or her medical care, or influence medical decision-making?

REFLECTIONS

ᐒ Have you ever had a physician inquire about your spirituality? If so, how did that affect you? If not, would this be something you would desire?

ᐒ What is your experience with asking spiritual questions?

🔖 Can you recall a patient whose religious beliefs significantly influenced medical care? What were the circumstances? What was your response?

NURSING'S APPROACH

There is considerable literature dealing with nursing's response to spiritual needs. As a group, nurses are more similar to patients in their religious beliefs and practices than are physicians.[12] Furthermore, it is part of nurses' heritage to integrate spirituality into the care they deliver. This response is supported by the American Nurses' Association Standards of Nursing Practice and the American Nurses' Association Code of Ethics for Nurses, documents that identify standards of practice and conduct for the nursing profession as a whole.

In addition, each of the specialty areas in nursing—psychiatric and mental health nursing, home care nursing, emergency nursing—have similar standards of practice. Each of these official documents recognizes the importance of assessing and meeting identified spiritual needs. Furthermore, the North American Nursing Diagnosis Association has identified "spiritual distress," "risk for spiritual distress," and "readiness for enhanced spiritual well-being" as acceptable diagnoses in identifying the focus of nursing care. The Nursing Interventions Classification identifies "religious ritual enhancement," "religious addiction prevention," and "spiritual support" as appropriate nursing interventions.[13] The Nursing Outcomes Classification includes "spiritual well-being" as an appropriate outcome of nursing intervention.[14]

So what is nursing's approach to assessing spiritual needs?

Because nurses see patients in many different settings and frequently have more extended contact with patients than many other healthcare professionals, they are encouraged to broaden their approach to assessing spirituality. Certainly, a structured spiritual assessment is necessary. Before we get to that, however, let's look at the other aspects that the nurse considers when evaluating a spiritual need. Nurses are educated to look at the patient's nonverbal as well as verbal behavior and to closely observe the environment for sources of information.

Following are the observations that are part of a spiritual assessment:[15]

Nonverbal Behavior

1. Observe affect. Does the patient's affect or attitude convey loneliness, depression, anger, agitation, or anxiety?

2. Observe behavior. Does the patient pray? Does the patient rely on religious reading material or other literature for solace?

Verbal Behavior

1. Does the patient seem to complain out of proportion to his or her illness?

2. Does the patient complain of sleeping problems?

3. Does the patient ask for unusually high doses of sedation or pain medication?

4. Does the patient refer to God in any way?

5. Does the patient talk about prayer, faith, hope, or anything of a religious nature?

6. Does the patient talk about church functions that are part of his or her life?

7. Does the patient express concern over the meaning and direction of life? Does the patient express concern over the impact of illness on the meaning of life?

Interpersonal Relationships

1. Does the patient have visitors, or does he or she spend visiting hours alone?

2. Does the patient have a supportive family? Friends? Members of his or her faith community?

3. How does the patient interact with you and other staff members?

Environment

1. Does the patient have a Bible or other religious reading material?

2. Does the patient wear religious medals or pins?

3. Does the patient have religious articles such as statues as part of his or her religious observances?

4. Has the patient received religious get-well cards? Does the patient use personal pictures, artwork, or music to keep his or her spirits up?

The observations made by a nurse require validation for their meaning. For example, a patient who is displaying signs of sadness, anger, agitation, or anxiety may be expressing an emotional problem, or he may be expressing a spiritual concern through emotional channels. The content of a patient's verbalizations also provides the nurse with insights about the patient's feelings and needs. For instance, do the patient's complaints seem disproportionate in relation to the severity of her illness? Does the patient make repeated requests for pain medication and sedation? Does the patient complain of sleeping difficulties? All these behaviors may indicate a physical need, but they also may provide clues that the patient is experiencing spiritual distress.

It is important to note whether the patient talks about God and in what ways the patient refers to God. Sometimes the patient may reveal the presence of a deep spiritual need by joking about "the Man upstairs" or other such lighthearted references to God. Patients may discuss serious issues like their own death with a gallows humor, another indication of spiritual need. Patients may talk openly about their faith, religious practices, beliefs, hope, forgiveness, or prayer, providing an opening to a deeper exploration of their spirituality.

Also worthy of observation are the quantity and, more importantly, the quality of interpersonal relationships in which the patient is involved. Does the patient have a supportive circle of family and friends that she can depend on for assistance? If the patient does not have a support system with which to interact and people in her life with whom to communicate love and concern, then the patient may also be experiencing a similar estrangement from God. After all, much of one's knowledge of God's love is derived from the quality of love that is exchanged with significant others.[16]

Additional observations include noting whether the patient has a

Bible, other religious reading material, or religious objects such as medals, pins, a prayer shawl, a mezuzah, or a rosary or other prayer beads, in her environment. These objects may mean nothing at all to the patient, or they may have important spiritual significance.

An adequate assessment also involves interviewing the patient. Most nursing assessments start by asking, What is your faith tradition? and, Would you like me to contact someone in your faith community? These questions are a beginning, but they are insufficient for eliciting a complete spiritual assessment.

Here are the areas to be covered in a spiritual assessment and questions that assist the nurse in completing this inquiry:[17]

Concept of God or Deity

1. Is religion or God important to you? If so, can you describe how?

2. Is prayer helpful to you? What happens when you pray?

3. Does God or a deity function in your personal life? If yes, can you describe how?

4. How would your describe God or this deity?

Sources of Strength and Hope

1. Who is the most important person to you?

2. To whom do you turn when you need help? Are they available?

3. In what ways do they help?

4. What is your source of strength and hope?

5. What helps you the most when you are afraid or need help?

Religious Practices

1. Do you feel your faith or religion is helpful to you? If yes, could you tell me how?

2. Are there any religious practices that are important to you?

3. Has being sick (or what has happened to you) made any difference in your practice of praying? Your religious practices?

Relation between Spiritual Beliefs and Health

1. What has bothered you the most about being sick (or what is happening to you)?

2. What do you think is going to happen to you?

3. Has being sick (or what has happened to you) made any difference in your feelings about God or the practice of your faith?

4. Is there anything that is especially frightening or meaningful to you now?

Need for Spiritual Assistance

1. Is there anything that I can do to support you spiritually?

2. Would you want someone to pray for you? With you?

3. Would you like me to call the chaplain? Your pastor? Your priest? Your rabbi? Your imam? Your faith community?

Medicine and nursing offer approaches to eliciting the spiritual story that are useful to other healthcare professionals and could certainly be adapted to different clinical settings. What is important is that the spiritual conversation takes place, and that the findings are communicated to the healthcare team in a manner that alerts others to the patient's spiritual needs so they can think of ways to assist the patient in this journey—but without unnecessarily alarming the patient, who might perceive the asking of spiritual questions as a signal that his illness is incurable or her condition is much worse than expected. Appendix B includes additional assessment resources.

REFLECTIONS

❧ Can you think of a situation where you became aware of a spiritual need by observing a patient's nonverbal behavior? What were the circumstances? How did you validate your observations?

❧ What kind of signals do you give to others regarding your own spirituality or religious beliefs/practices?

❧ How would you react if a patient requested that you pray with her? Read Scripture?

◈ Once you have determined that a patient is experiencing a spiritual need, what avenues are open to you for assisting the patient?

RESPONDING TO SPIRITUAL NEEDS

Once you have completed a spiritual history/assessment, what do you do with the information? Let's start with what you don't do: You don't proselytize, preach, or demean the beliefs of the patient.

There are three major categories of interventions—ministry of presence, ministry of word, and ministry of action. In reality these ministries overlap and sustain each other, but for the purpose of discussion we will examine each independently.

Ministry of Presence

Ministry of presence requires more than just showing up when someone is sick or standing by the bedside, although these actions are important. To fully demonstrate the ministry of presence, we need to be active listeners, to be empathetic, vulnerable, humble, and committed.[18]

Active listening is a learned skill that involves not just hearing the words being spoken but also those that are not spoken. Frequently people only hint at their real concerns, and openly reveal them only when we go beyond their words to their feelings and the deeper meaning behind their communication. This requires that we develop sensitivity to the barriers we set up to active listening. Those barriers include our own anxiety and personal defenses, judgments about patients and their behaviors, and the fact that words can have many meanings, and differing interpretations can build walls instead of bridges.

Anxiety makes us focus more on ourselves than on the other person. There are many reasons for anxiety, and none of us is immune to it. Maybe it has just been a terrible day. The car wouldn't start, traffic was unbelievably heavy, the day began with an angry complaint from a patient, and so on. This is probably not the best time to deal with the spirituality of another. It is important that we manage our own anxiety, perhaps drawing on personal spiritual resources, in order to be present to another.

Related to anxiety is our need to use our personal defenses to block communication. Sometimes patients or families say things that deeply offend us. We feel as if something we value is under attack, and instead of listening, we defend our position. In so doing we effectively place an impenetrable barrier between us and the very person to whom we are called to minister.

Judging another's behavior is another major barrier to active listening. Sometimes a patient's life choices are in direct contradiction to our beliefs and values, and we might be tempted to conclude that his suffering is deserved. If we remain in judgment, however, we cannot help the patient—in fact, we will be subjecting the patient to spiritual abuse. It is necessary to suspend judgment and try to see beyond the facts, the behaviors, and the lifestyle choices to where hurt lives. Only then can we minister.

Lastly, we need to be aware that word meanings differ from person to person. Words can be laden with emotional weight that influences a person's response. For instance, the word *spirituality* might engender very different responses from different people.

Empathy, the next component of presence, involves using our minds and hearts to understand a person's story. It is necessary for us to connect with the pain of another, to feel the situation as that person feels it, otherwise we will remain aloof and disconnected. Once we feel the pain, we need to use our minds to understand objectively what the patient is describing and to offer assistance. Giving only a heart response is not empathy, it is sympathy. Sympathy not only encourages the person to remain in a place of pain, but it emotionally immobilizes us, and we are unable to assist the person to move to a better place. Giving only a mind response is cold, impersonal, and disinterested and will make the patient feel uncared about and misunderstood. The combination of heart and mind in the form of empathy is what the patient needs.

To be empathetic, we must be *vulnerable*. When we open ourselves up to others, we feel their pain; we take a chance of being rejected and criticized. Making ourselves available to others is draining. The rewards, however, are great—the possibility of joy and knowing that we have made a difference in the life of another awaits those who are willing to be vulnerable.

Humility is the next component of a ministry of presence, and it involves recognizing our strengths and limitations. Humility involves the realization that we are not the only one who might be able to assist the patient, and that we alone are not the sole source of ministry. Humility allows us to be open to learn from those to whom we provide care.

Commitment, the last aspect of the ministry of presence, involves our willingness to maintain the relationship as long as the person requires spiritual support, even when the commitment costs us.[19] The ministry of presence is what God provides each of us, and we have the responsibility and privilege of extending that to God's people. There are no denominational boundaries on this type of ministry; it is open to everyone, and from it everyone can benefit. "David's Story" is an example of the ministry of presence.

DAVID'S STORY

I was a psychiatric homecare nurse, and I received a referral to see David, an elderly man who had been diagnosed with psychosis. I had provided care to many people with that diagnosis, so I believed that I knew what to expect. Wow, was I surprised. During my initial nursing assessment, I began to do a spiritual assessment, and I thought that I had opened Pandora's box. David spewed out such hatred toward God, anything religious, anyone religious, the Bible, and all Christian beliefs. He told me that there was no personal God, but that he knew there was a personal devil. His anger was so powerful it pushed me back in my chair. Over the years I have worked hard to control my outward reactions, but inside I was churning. David had gotten to me. The best that I could manage was to be quiet. I reacted inside with disgust. He was being blasphemous. I wanted to set him straight. Thank God I didn't. I remained quiet and tried to listen.

After I left him and collected my thoughts, I tried to figure out what had taken place. He clearly touched areas of my heart where I felt defensive. I wasn't able to hear him, and I knew that if I were going to help him, I had to figure out a way of dealing with myself before I would be able to deal with David. I thought about him all week. I prayed that God would let me see David as God saw him, and I asked God to help me really listen to what David was telling me.

The next week I went to see David again, and after we covered whether he had taken his medications and reviewed his week, I told him I was intrigued by his views on religion and God and asked if we could revisit this area. It didn't take much to get him started, but this time it was different. I was able to really listen to him. I suspended my judgment and remained calm inside. I asked him where these views came from.

Then he told me his story. His dad had forced him to go to Mass every Sunday. However, his father was certainly not a religious person. He was an abusive alcoholic. Several times a week he would return home stoned drunk after drinking until the wee hours of the morning. He would come into David's room, kneel on his bed, and, with a lit cigarette dangling from his mouth and dropping ashes on David, he would beat his son. His abuse was not limited to physical beatings but also included verbal berating. David's life was a living hell—beatings at night and verbal tirades during the day. David heard that he was a bad boy, that he was one of God's mistakes, and that surely he would burn in hell. All this from a father who never missed Mass and insisted that David attend as well!

All of my judgment from the week before melted away, and in its place was incredible compassion for this man. So many of us first experience God's love from our parents—David had experienced something very different. The amount of pain that he felt was overwhelming. I knew that I alone could not bring him healing, but God working through me could do amazing things.

This day was the beginning of my relationship with David. I continued to work with him for many months. The improvement was dramatic. Although he would never be an "easy person," he moved to a much more peaceful place, and I believe that his change started when I was able to really listen to him, to feel his pain, to be present to him, and to ask for God's help in working with David.

—Verna Benner Carson

REFLECTIONS

❧ What is your experience with providing presence to others?

❧ What is your experience with receiving presence from others? How did this help you (or not) spiritually?

❧ Can you think of some examples when you were able to engage in active listening? Did you find it difficult? Why? What were the results?

❧ What happens to you when another person actively listens to you?

❧ Can you think of patient/family situations where you could see that your ability to be empathetic, vulnerable, humble, and committed resulted in spiritual well-being for those to whom you ministered? What was the benefit to you?

❧ Can you think of patient/family situations where you were unable to be empathetic, vulnerable, humble, and committed—where, in other words, you were not present to them? How were the outcomes of those situations different from when you were able to be present?

Ministry of Word

The ministry of word aspect of spiritual care requires great sensitivity to the patient's belief system. Words are incredibly powerful. They can be life-giving or they can be destructive, so care must be used in choosing what to say. Included in this ministry are: (1) a willingness to discuss spiritual/religious issues; (2) verbal support and encouragement of spiritual beliefs; (3) making a referral to a chaplain; (4) using scripture or other religious literature; and (5) using prayer.

The act of taking a spiritual history or assessment is really the first aspect of this form of caring. The very act of engaging in a conversation about spirituality conveys to the patient and family that we are *willing to discuss spiritual/religious beliefs and issues.* This initial spiritual conversation may very well lead to other opportunities to talk about the impact of these spiritual matters on the patient's current health situation—issues such as: (1) how will the patient cope, (2) what impact will this health crisis have on the patient's sense of purpose and meaning in life, (3) what adaptations or changes need to be made to accommodate the current health problem, and (4) what difficult choices face the patient/family? Every one of these questions is spiritual in nature. We may not have the answers, nor is it necessary that we have the answers. In fact, even if we believe we have the answers, it is usually best to encourage the patient and family to talk openly about these issues until they are able to arrive at their own answers.

Supporting and encouraging the patient's religious and spiritual views is another aspect of ministry of the word. This support must always be patient centered—that is, we are not introducing our own beliefs but are encouraging the beliefs and practices that bring comfort to the patient. Healthcare providers must exercise care to avoid even a hint of coercion in this area. Our job is to provide care, and that involves spiritual care, but we are not to preach. We might feel more at ease supporting beliefs and practices when the patient's belief system is either the same as our own or similar. When the patient expresses beliefs that seem strange and unfamiliar to us, however, we need to ask for further clarification, to be respectful, and to encourage the patient's personal reflection.

Making a referral to a chaplain or the patient's own spiritual leader is the third aspect of ministry of the word. Most healthcare providers lack the expertise to answer theological questions or perform specific religious rites or rituals. Sometimes the patient reveals the presence of a spiritual need but feels more at ease discussing it with a member of the clergy. At other times, the healthcare professional lacks comfort intervening in spiritual issues or lacks the training and may refer these needs to the clergy. Whatever the reason, the referral should be discussed with the patient and the patient's wishes respected.

Use of scripture or other religious literature is the fourth component of the ministry of the word. This intervention requires great sensitivity to the cues from the patient, and the decision to use it must flow from the spiritual assessment. It is certainly appropriate for the healthcare provider to inquire if the patient has a special passage or reading and to ascertain the reason for its specialness. In this case, the healthcare provider is invoking something that already has personal meaning for the patient and may indeed serve as a support for the patient. If the patient indicates that reading or discussing scripture would be helpful, it is appropriate to honor the patient's requests.

Prayer is the fifth component of a ministry of the word. It is a powerful intervention and certainly has a place in healthcare. Prayer is described in many different ways. The writings of the great spiritual leaders of all traditions of faith acknowledge the centrality of prayer to a life with God. Prayer is an invitation to the Divine to enter into our lives in an active way. Prayer builds a bridge between individuals and their God.[20] Prayer is the communication of the soul reaching out to a personal God and forming a relationship. Through this relationship the individual communicates needs, feelings, fears, love, adoration, and awe to the Creator. In return, the person is graced with a sense of God's presence and abiding love.

Illness can interfere with an individual's ability to pray. Feelings such as isolation, fear, guilt, grief, and anxiety can flow from the illness experience. These feelings can be barriers to relationships in general, and specifically to the relationship one has with God. Patients may feel that prayers will not come, that they feel cut off from God and unable to bridge the gap **Words are incredibly powerful. They can be life-giving or they can be destructive, so care must be used in choosing what to say.** between themselves and their Creator. At least one study has found that patients who feel this way have significantly worse future health outcomes, independent of their physical or emotional health.[21] The healthcare provider's offer to pray with or for a patient can break through that sense of isolation and allow the patient to feel the comfort of God's love through the healthcare provider.

A few caveats are necessary regarding the use of prayer. It should always be patient centered, and it should be something the patient desires. There should be a valid reason to pray. In addition, we must be certain, based on the spiritual assessment, that the patient will appreciate the offer of prayer. If the patient and healthcare provider are of different religious backgrounds, it is necessary to ask the patient how she prays. If the healthcare provider is not comfortable praying as the patient prays, an offer to pray silently while the patient prays out loud may be an adequate alternative. It is important to keep in mind that the purpose of prayer is to help the patient in her relationship with God (however the patient perceives God); the healthcare provider must therefore use an approach that brings the patient peace and does not create anxiety. In all situations the healthcare provider can pray silently for the patient.

Dr. Shahid Athar shares his experience with silent prayer:

After using all the necessary medicines, I found that patients' responses were not all the same. In some, the medicine worked, and in some it did not. Therefore, like a combination antibiotic or chemotherapy, I started to add prayer to my patient's treatment regimen, Muslims as well as non-Muslims. I never told them that I was praying, but after giving them medicine, I prayed for them by name, asking God to make my medicine effective, comfort their pain, and give each one healing through his or her own power of healing. I observed that this practice worked, but I do not know how.[22]

"Sandy's Story" is an example of praying with a patient.

SANDY'S STORY

Sandy had end-stage renal disease and had just been released from a long and torturous inpatient stay for treatment of sepsis. She was released with a permanent tracheostomy; she was blind because she had required 100 percent oxygen; and she had a painful and deep decubitus on her sacrum. Sandy was pretty much bed-bound. She was not in good shape. I was seeing her because she was incredibly depressed and angry—at God, her body, the world, and everyone who was healthy. She had every right to be angry. I worked with her for over a year. Early on I learned that we shared the same faith and had attended the same Catholic school, and our birthdays were only a day apart. I was the older one—and, fortunately for me, the healthier one.

Completing the assessment was a challenge, because she had difficulty communicating. Either she covered her tracheostomy to answer my questions, or she wrote on a small blackboard she kept by the bedside. We established that she was a praying person and that prayer was something that she wanted from me. I asked her how she wanted me to pray—using a formal prayer, like the Lord's Prayer, or an informal conversational prayer. She chose the informal conversational approach. At the end of every visit I would ask her what she wanted me to pray. I would then hold her hand and speak her prayer to God. I always added my own prayer that God give her peace and that Sandy would know God's love and feel God's presence.

She made great progress—I was able to get her out of bed and seated at a piano in her living room. If I placed her hands on the keys of the piano and called out the keys, she could play simple melodies. This gave her great joy! Then the unthinkable happened—she became septic again and was readmitted to the hospital. When she was discharged, I resumed psychiatric home care for her. If I thought she had been angry before, she was full of rage now and wanted to die. Prayer was again an important part of what I did for Sandy—if I forgot she would write on her blackboard, in large letters, PRAY! She wrote with such force that on a few occasions she shattered the chalk.

Nothing I did seemed to help her. I felt useless. Before going into her house, there were many times when I would sit in my car trying to find the courage to make the visit and praying hard for direction. On one such occasion, I was telling the Lord that I had nothing left to give Sandy when I had a strong sense of the Lord's direction: although I was feeling that I had nothing left, the Lord had plenty more for her, and I needed to continue to pray. I made myself go into her home that morning and many mornings afterwards. Sandy finally made the decision to end her dialysis. I believe that the prayers we shared helped her reach a place of peace where she was able to make this decision.

—Verna Benner Carson

REFLECTIONS

🙣 Have you ever used the ministry of word to assist a patient and/or family in spiritual distress? What were the circumstances? What was the outcome?

🙣 What would you do if the patient's religious beliefs were in conflict with medical treatment?

🙣 Have you ever prayed with a patient? How did that come about? What were the circumstances?

🙣 Has a healthcare provider ever ministered to you through words? Has a healthcare provider ever prayed with you? How did that affect you?

Ministry of Action

Ministry of action refers, quite simply, to how you do what you do. The simplest acts are capable of conveying a powerful message of love.

Marilyn Bullock shares a story of working in a long-term-care facility:

There was a nun at the far end of our unit; I didn't usually take care of her. No one wanted to take care of her. Everyone thought she was going to die, and she wasn't the easiest person—kind of crotchety and grouchy. Anyway, one day we were short staffed, and I was asked to take Sister's medicine to her. I was told to take along applesauce to make it easier for her to take her pills. I did that, and when I was done, I offered her a glass of cold water, for which she seemed grateful. I never took care of her again. Two years later, I saw this very tiny nun walking toward our nurse's station—it was Sister. She said, "I know that voice! Where is she?" (I have a slight Boston accent, or so I'm told.) Sister came up to me and hugged me. She said, "You gave me the glass of cold water. That was the kindest thing anyone did for me, and I have never forgotten it." Can you believe a glass of water could be that powerful?

Another story comes from nurse Beatrice Rosen:

I remember while working in a homecare environment, I had a weekend assignment to do a dressing change for an elderly man. He had been homeless and had been given an apartment by the state. He had just moved in. It was a very hot day—probably close to 100 degrees. The apartment was oppressive, the refrigerator didn't work, and there was no fan available. He didn't have shoes or socks. He was a diabetic. I remember doing the dressing change, making sure he had his medications, and addressing his medical needs. After the day was done, he remained in my heart. With my husband's help, we returned to his apartment with food, a newspaper, shoes and socks, and a fan in tow. For us these were small offerings—for him they were a "God"-send.

Our last story comes from internist Julie Steiner:

I took care of an elderly woman who had had lung cancer surgery and had never fully recovered, despite our best efforts medically. I knew she was suffering in multiple ways—family and financial issues were problems, as well as her deteriorating medical condition. Fortunately, I am in a practice associated with a hospital system that has a charity program, which I had her enrolled in. Then I saw her every week until she passed away. Being available to her was a blessing to me and to her. I was so glad I could cut through the financial and administrative red tape and just spend time with her, helping her in whatever way that I could.

Acts of love come packaged in many ways, and they don't always take a lot of time. We need to continue to be aware that the mighty as well as the tiny things that we do for someone each have the potential to convey love—and at the heart of spiritual care is a ministry of love.

REFLECTIONS

☙ Can you remember being touched by a small act of kindness? What impact did that have on you?

☙ How can you minister to your patients through your actions? How do your actions convey love and compassion?

SPIRITUAL CARE AND THE HEALTHCARE TEAM

We have addressed the roles of the physician and nurse, but what about other members of the team? How do each of the other healthcare providers—social workers, therapists, nursing assistants, counselors, and chaplains—fit into the picture of providing spiritual care?

Ideally, the physician would begin the process with a spiritual history documented in the patient's chart; the nurse would review this history and ask the patient only spiritual questions that might have bearing on nursing care. The nurse and/or social worker would then assist to mobilize spiritual resources (including a visit with the chaplain, the patient's clergy or parish nurse, and/or members of the patient's faith community) to help the patient cope with illness during hospitalization and after discharge. A care conference would be held to discuss the spiritual needs of the patient, and a plan for meeting these needs would be drawn up. Individual providers on the team would be assigned roles in this care as appropriate.

We have examined how we engage in a spiritual conversation with a patient. We have looked at the approaches used by medicine and nursing to collect critical spiritual information. We have described the ways to intervene to meet spiritual needs. In the next chapter, we explore what spiritual care looks like in specific situations, such as when a patient is dying, dealing with a chronic illness, or suffering with a psychiatric illness.

[6]

Giving Spiritual Care
The Patient with Chronic Illness and Pain

Day by day
Day by day
O dear Lord
Three things I pray
To see thee more clearly
To love thee more dearly
To follow thee more nearly
Day by day
Day by day by day . . .

—Godspell

The words from the musical *Godspell* speak directly to all of us called to act as ministers of healthcare. To see God in those that we serve, to love them, and to follow God's direction in providing care—this is our mission. Ideally, this is what we do with all patients. There are certain patients, however, in whom the presence of spiritual needs should always be assumed. Then our spiritual conversations serve to provide us clear direction in meeting these needs.

We posed the following question to the participants in our healthcare survey: In the literature, there are a number of specific patient situations where spirituality and/or religious belief and practices influence not only the patient's needs but also the healthcare provider's response to these needs. These include patients dealing with chronic illnesses and pain, living with AIDS, those who are dying, those who are grieving, suffering from psychiatric illness, and declining from Alzheimer's and other dementias. Can you provide an example(s) where you identified a patient or family's spiritual and/or religious needs and responded out of your own spirituality?

Our participants provided us with many examples of patient situations beyond what we asked. Let's examine the responses we received, beginning in this chapter with a close look at patients with chronic illness and pain. In a sense, the spiritual care to these patients provides a model for other patient situations—each of which are often associated with chronicity and/or pain.

Chronic illnesses and pain impose multiple challenges, including alteration in self-perception and self-control, the need to grieve over a long period of time, the need to readapt to the limitations imposed by the illness, the need to deal with the uneasy responses of others, and the need to come to terms with significant spiritual issues.[1] These patients may be seen frequently over a long period by the same healthcare provider or a group of providers. It is important for us to realize that our relationship(s) with these patients can be a vehicle for their healing and wholeness. We have a responsibility to respond not only to the immediate physical distress resulting from the chronic illness, but also to the whole gamut of spiritual implications that compose the picture of chronic illness.

SELF-PERCEPTION AND SELF-CONTROL

Many patients express a sense of being trapped in a body that fails them daily. They have so much on the inside that they want and are ready to accomplish but are unable to accomplish because of physical limitations imposed by the illness. Their sense of self-control is damaged as well. Sometimes the pain and disability that accompany the illness strip the person of his or her sense of control. It is important, as much as possible, for people with chronic illnesses to believe that they are *in control of* the pain and disability and not *controlled by* the pain and disability.

GRIEF

Grief is another issue confronting those who live with chronic illness. It is different from the grief experienced after a death, which generally is time limited. The losses that accompany chronic illness do not occur all at once; instead, there is a continual process of losing that may continue throughout the person's lifetime, and so the grieving is also extended. New exacerbations of an old illness may result in increased loss of function and pain. Many times the grief becomes a chronic sorrow not easily worked through. Engle is credited with identifying the stages of grieving associated with death.[2] Crate adapted Engel's stages to look at the grieving associated with chronic illness.[3] Table 3 compares the grieving process associated with death to a similar process of adaptation in chronic illness.

READAPTATION

Readaptation, according to Feldman, "is coming to terms existentially with the reality of chronic illness as a state of being, discarding both false hope and destructive hopelessness, and restructuring the environment in which one must now function."[4] What is required for readaptation is the development of practical skills that enhance life and decrease destructive stress.

Everyone is confronted with stress. The person with a chronic illness, however, is constantly stressed, not only by the illness itself but also by efforts required to maintain some semblance of a normal lifestyle. Even more than the average person, people who live with chronic illness need internal emotional and spiritual resources to manage stress on a daily basis. Readaptation also involves achieving a healthy balance between

TABLE 3. Grieving Process and Adaptation to Chronic Illness

Engel's Process of Grieving	*Crate's Stages of Adaptation*
Shock and disbelief: "No, it can't be" refusal to accept fact	Disbelief: denial of threatening condition to protect self; "I don't have it"
Developing awareness: reality begins to penetrate consciousness	Developing awareness: uses anger as a defense against dependency or guilt about being sick
Restitution: the work of mourning, identification with the loss	Reorganization: accepts illness and/or increased dependence; reorganizes relationships with family and friends to accommodate illness
Resolution: dealing with void, preoccupation with loss	Idealization: psychic dependence on loss decreases; allows a reinterest in life to occur
Adaptation	Resolution: acknowledges changes in how sees self; identification with others with same problem
Identity: defines self as an individual who is changing but worthwhile	Adaptation: able to live with illness; able to acknowledge self as having limits and needing to live differently

Taken from R. I. Stoll, "Spirituality and Chronic Illness," 189.

retaining self-control over daily activities and accepting assistance when help is needed to have personal needs met. This balance comes from a positive self-image as well as from trust in the acceptance and respect of others. People with chronic illness usually have to "grow into" this balance—it doesn't just happen.[5]

SOCIAL RESPONSES

Those with chronic illnesses also elicit difficult responses from others. People can be sympathetic when a person is acutely ill, but there is usually an expectation of healing and getting better. When the illness lingers and waxes and wanes in its effects on the person's life, others neither understand nor know how to respond in a helpful manner. They may avoid the person with a chronic illness or ignore the presence and impact of the illness, not knowing what to say or how to be helpful; or worse, they may accuse the person of exaggerating the symptoms.

When the illness lingers and waxes and wanes in its effects on the person's life, others neither understand nor know how to respond in a helpful manner.

This only increases the sense of isolation felt by those dealing with chronic illnesses and pain. Even healthcare providers are guilty of being less than helpful to those with chronic illness. Sometimes these patients are put on the defensive and made to feel as if they are complainers when they don't fully respond to the interventions of the healthcare provider or team.

SPIRITUAL RESOURCES

Medical research clearly shows that patients find comfort through spiritual beliefs and practices and are better able to cope when they have an integrated personal religious motivation that provides hope and meaning in life and illness.[6] Stoll identifies three spiritual beliefs that are significant resources in learning to live with chronic illness and pain: trust, hope, and courage.[7]

Trust

Those who suffer with the uncertainties of a chronic illness, who struggle through days of exhaustion where every effort seems to require more energy and stamina than is available, who fight the temptation to give in to self-pity and despair, desperately need someone or something to hold onto and to trust. As Stoll puts it, "Sufferers need to experience something or someone that can infuse them with the almost supernatural energy to resist the temptation to retreat, remembering 'there are better days.'"[8] The words of the Psalmist David speak to his recognition that he could hold onto God: "Even though I walk through the valley of the shadow of death, I will fear no evil for you are with me, your rod and your staff they comfort me" (Psalm 23).[9]

Many who are confronted with chronic illness hold onto the belief that God is always with them. Over 40 percent of medical inpatients in some areas of the country indicate that such beliefs are their most important source of comfort (more important than any other factor in helping them cope).[10] Healthcare providers must also be concerned with creating trust. We should be seen as people whom the patient can hold onto and trust. It is essential, therefore, that we be honest with patients and not encourage illusions or avoid difficult possibilities.

Leon illustrates how important trust in God can be to a patient.

LEON'S TRUST IN GOD

Leon was a thirty-five-year-old man with chronic paranoid schizophrenia. I received a referral to see him from the Maryland Psychiatric Research Center, where Leon had enrolled in a Clozaril research study. My role was to teach him about the medication, assess the effectiveness of the medication and the presence of side effects, encourage him to return weekly to the research center for blood tests, and generally to provide him with psychotherapeutic support while he was in the study.

When I met Leon, he told me that in addition to participating in the study, he had enrolled in a work-study program at one of the local community colleges, where he would be taking sixteen credit hours of study while working twenty hours per week. I told him that since he didn't know how he would respond to the medication change (prior to the study he required Prolixin Decanoate as well as oral DProlixin and was still bothered by voices), this sounded like a recipe for failure. He told me that I didn't really understand and that he viewed the work-study program as his last chance to make something of his life.

He had experienced his first symptoms of schizophrenia when he was a freshman in college. All his friends who had been in school with him at that time were now married with families and careers. He said, "Where am I? I am a chronic schizophrenic; I have been in every state hospital in Maryland; I have been arrested more times than I can remember because when I am sick, I am pretty scary to people. This might be my last chance." This is a hard position to argue with—Leon was sharing the meaning that schizophrenia had in his life.

Over the next few weeks, it was obvious that Leon was not receiving Clozaril. Not only was he free of the side effects of Clozaril, but more importantly, he was increasingly bothered by voices. One day I came for the home-

care visit, and Leon was visibly distraught. When I asked what the problem was, Leon told me that before class this day, some of the students were gathered outside of the classroom, laughing and talking. One of the students glanced his way as she laughed. Immediately he began to hear his voices telling him, "They know you're crazy—they're saying you're dangerous—they don't want to be around you."

When I asked Leon how he had coped with this, he told me that during class it had taken an enormous amount of effort to tell himself to ignore the voices, that they were not real. I then asked him how he planned to go back to class tomorrow. He told me that he wasn't sure how he would handle class, but tonight he would do what he did every night of his life— "whether I am crazy or well." When I asked what that was, he told me that he prayed and read Scripture. I asked if he had a favorite Scripture passage, and he began to recite Psalm 23. I asked him what significance this Scripture passage had for him. He told me it reminded him that he was never alone. He said, "I never pray that God heals my schizophrenia. I'm sure I am going to die a schizophrenic. What I pray for is that God walks with me though all of it—the good times and the bad." I left Leon feeling very humbled by the depth of his trust and faith in God.

—Verna Benner Carson

Hope

People feel hopeful when they can trust that outside help is available and reliable. Invariably, the trustworthy sources of help are significant spiritual and human relationships. Hope is the sense that the individual's resources, including significant others and a loving, faithful God, are able and willing to consistently provide the needed support. The experience of hope encourages the individual to believe "I am not alone," "There is a way through," "The way may be difficult, but not impossible." When people are struggling with their illness or a change forced upon them by the illness, and they receive such a message of hope, they experience renewed vitality, strength, and the courage to persevere. As healthcare providers, we can accept

> Hope is the sense that the individual's resources, including significant others and a loving, faithful God, are able and willing to consistently provide the needed support.

the illness while always holding out hope that it is not necessary to accept the limitations that the illness seems to imply.

Courage

Courage and perseverance are closely related to hope. Stedman offers this description of courage: "the ability to abide under, to stay under the pressure . . . to hang in there . . . to develop the quality of steadiness and peace."[11] Courage is needed to persevere in the face of incredible odds. To be a courageous person does not preclude the presence of fear; rather, courage speaks to the ability to transcend one's fears, to choose to confront what needs to be done, to take pleasure in the joys that are still available, and to consciously avoid worrying and wishing for a potentially unattainable outcome. Courage and perseverance do not come easily but are forged out of the furnace of suffering. As healthcare providers, we can encourage perseverance; we can share stories of others who have persevered through courage; we can affirm the courageous acts and attitudes we see in patients and families.

REFLECTIONS

- Think about your experiences working with patients who suffered from chronic illness. What were the most difficult challenges faced by these patients? In what ways were you able to provide assistance?
- Can you think of an example of a patient displaying courage and perseverance in the face of a chronic illness? What were the circumstances? How did this affect you?
- What are the issues that challenge hope and trust in patients who are dealing with chronic illness? What is your role in supporting hope and trust?
- Do you or does someone you love suffer from a chronic illness? If so, how has this personal experience affected your practice? What spiritual beliefs serve as resources to you?

COPING RESPONSES

There are a number of practical coping strategies used by those who deal with chronic illness and pain. These include (1) prayer, (2) use of the "Faith Factor" with the Relaxation Response, (3) humor, (4) music and bibliotherapy, (5) keeping a journal, and (6) reaching out to others. Sharing information about these coping skills is an important aspect of spiritual care.

Prayer

People with chronic illness use prayer to present their needs to God, to express their thankfulness, and to confess their dependency on a God whose strength is infinite. Prayer provides tremendous comfort to someone who daily experiences the finiteness of personal strength and resources. Prayer reflects an intimate relationship with a God that is loving and accepting; it can be an expression of hope that God will be and is reliable. Prayer also provides an outlet for anger and confusion toward a God who is seen as the source of pain, suffering, and loss.

With all these benefits in mind, it is important to recognize that prayer is not always easy for someone with a chronic illness. Sometimes the illness saps energy and mental concentration to such a degree that only the briefest entreaty to God is possible. At such times the prayers of a supportive person, a prayer network, or shared prayer with the suffering individual can fill the gap between the individual and God. As healthcare providers, we cannot prescribe prayer unless we know through our spiritual history that this is something the patient values. As an educational intervention, however, we might be able to share research findings about the value of prayer without any hint of coercion or proselytizing on our part.

The "Faith Factor" with the Relaxation Response

Experiencing stress and anxiety is part of living with chronic illness. It is important that patients learn how to relax and release the stress they feel. Dr. Herbert Benson describes the effectiveness of the faith factor as an additive to one's use of the relaxation technique: "The combination of a Relaxation-Response technique with the individual's belief system is what I call the 'Faith Factor' . . . two powerful but familiar vehicles are combined: (1) meditation and (2) a deeply held set of philosophical or religious beliefs."[12]

Dr. Benson is not promoting one religious faith over another. In fact, he is not promoting religion. He contends, however, that it does matter what we believe. It is out of our conviction about the unique power of faith that we ignite quantifiable, scientifically measurable physiological changes that serve to disrupt the inner anxiety cycle. "It allows your mind to 'settle down,'" says Benson, "and move into more productive thought patterns."[13] Dr. Benson provides examples of phrases from the Christian and Jewish traditions, the Hindu and Buddhist traditions, and the Muslim tradition to be used along with relaxation.

Humor

Laughter has the power to bring healing to body, mind, and spirit and to allow the suffering person to transcend—if only for a moment—the limitations imposed by pain and illness. Keeping a folder of humorous stories, jokes, and funny anecdotes is a useful strategy for patients coping with chronic illness. Asking patients about the last time they had a good belly laugh opens the door to a discussion about the therapeutic value of humor. Finding humorous Web sites might be a beneficial activity for someone who is homebound and dealing with a chronic illness. The discovered jokes, stories, and anecdotes could be shared with others as well as providing benefit to the searcher.

Music and Bibliotherapy

Music feeds the soul by providing both an emotional and a spiritual release. Music can relax and refresh the body. Some chronically ill persons, when asked how they coped with suffering, reported that they listened to music.[14]

A story of a nurse who provided care using her love of singing comes from Amy Pollman.

I was visiting a patient in her home for treatment of severe depression. I learned that her husband was also very ill; he was suffering from asbestosis. My patient

Faith-Related Words and Phrases to Be Used with the Relaxation Response

୧ଳ

For Roman Catholic and Other Christian Traditions
Variations on the Lord's Prayer: "Our Father who art in heaven," or "Hallowed be Thy Name"

Phrases from the Hail Mary: "Hail Mary, full of grace"

A phrase from Mary's Magnificat, Luke 1:46–55: "My soul magnifies the Lord"

୧ଳ

For Protestants
Psalm 23: "The Lord is my shepherd"

Psalm 100: "Make a joyful noise unto the Lord"

Jesus' teachings or word: "My peace I give unto you" (John 4:27), "Love one another" (John 15:12), or "I am the Way, the Truth, and the Life" (John 14:6)

Other meaningful passages from the New Testament, such as "Thy peace which passes . . . understanding" (Phil. 4:7), or "We have the mind of Christ" (1 Cor. 2:16)

୧ଳ

For Jews
The Hebrew word for "peace": *Shalom*

The Hebrew word for "one": *Echod*

Passages from the Old Testament, such as "You shall love your neighbor" (Lev. 19:18), or "God said, 'Let there be light'" (Gen. 1:3)

Phrases that conform to King David's practice of meditating on God's promises, precepts, law, works, wonders, name, and decrees

୧ଳ

For Muslims
The word for "God," Allah; "The Lord is wondrous, kind"

Adahum, "one God," the words of the first Muslim who called the faithful to prayer

୧ଳ

For Hindus and Buddhists
The Bhagavad-Gita, the preeminent Hindu scripture, says, "Joy is inward"

Mahatma Gandhi said, "Turn the spotlight inward"

Part of a favorite invocation of Hindu priests, "Thou art everywhere" and "Thou art without form"

Buddhist literature contains phrases like these: "Life is a journey" and "I surrender indifferently"

Adapted from Herbert Benson, *Beyond the Relaxation Response.*

*got better and I discharged her, but my concern about her continued because I
knew her husband's prognosis was very poor. After the discharge, I continued to
call the patient to check on her and periodically stopped by to see her. In one of
my telephone calls, I learned that the woman's husband had just died, and I
offered to visit the patient's home to offer comfort. I wanted to do something to
make her feel better, so I brought along a musical accompaniment tape. While I
was in the home I sang a song entitled, "Friends in High Places." This was so
comforting to my patient. She asked that I sing this at her husband's funeral,
which I did.*

Bibliotherapy means purposeful reading that allows people to broaden their horizons, learn from others, or experience catharsis. Reading not only provides a useful and enjoyable pastime, it provides wisdom, comfort, insight, guidance, inspiration, and patience as we hear our own experiences reflected in the writings of another.[15] In addition, religious writings may support faith and courage.

As healthcare providers, we need to encourage listening to music and reading a good book. In fact, it is helpful to share with patients music or reading material that we have found particularly soothing, refreshing, stimulating, or in some way enlightening to us.

Reaching Out to Others

It is easy to fall into a trap of despair, believing that chronic illness and pain have placed a huge roadblock in the way of creativity and reaching out. It is sometimes out of this pain, however, that inspiration is born. Chronic illnesses do not end a life; they may lead to a slower pace and even demand that new priorities be established, but they do not signal the end. Many people find that reaching out to others is the best medicine. Reaching out shifts the focus away from self and personal pain to the needs of others—and it just plain feels good!

For example, a homebound elderly woman with severe arthritis sends greeting cards to other shut-ins within her church community. A wheelchair-bound woman with multiple sclerosis mans the telephones to organize the volunteer network at her church. These activities not only benefit others, but they give meaning and purpose to a life in

---

Contributions of People with Chronic Illness

❧

Emily Dickinson produced beautiful poetry despite her poor health and a life of seclusion.

❧

Henri Matisse took up painting as a distraction while convalescing from a serious illness.

❧

Robert Louis Stevenson suffered with severe pulmonary disease from birth; he wrote *Treasure Island, Dr. Jekyll and Mr. Hyde,* and *Kidnapped* while living in the shadow of death.

❧

Franklin Delano Roosevelt, thirty-second president of the United States, the only president elected to four terms in office, was a polio survivor.

❧

Ann Ruth, a quadriplegic, is an artist and president of the Ann Ruth Greeting Card Company. She paints by holding the brush in her teeth.

❧

Wendy Whiting, restricted to a wheelchair due to spastic cerebral palsy, choreographs ballets. Although she cannot perform, she has dancers who help her make her vision a reality.

E. G. Wheeler and J. Dace-Lombard, *Living Creatively with Chronic Illness*

---

which meaning and purpose have been brought into question because of the limitations imposed by chronic illness. As healthcare providers encounter patients who feel full of despair, believing they have no purpose, we need to provide them an alternate view of what their lives could be like. Sharing stories of people who found their talents and gifts and made a difference in the world *after* being diagnosed with chronic illness[16] is a powerful intervention, as long as we don't make the patients feel as though they are being compared—which could further deflate their sense of self-esteem.

Journaling

The practice of keeping a journal can serve many purposes. Recording feelings, struggles, and prayers can release pent-up emotions, open the door to new ways of thinking, renew the spirit, and build a storehouse of memories. Journaling is a conversation with self that helps to clarify thoughts and feelings; doubt and anger may be released and faith affirmed. The Psalms, which many people find so comforting, are in reality David's journal cataloging the ups and downs of his spiritual journey.

Even the medical literature documents the benefits of journaling. The results of a randomized clinical trial of journaling, conducted in patients with asthma or rheumatoid arthritis, was published in the *Journal of the American Medical Association* in 1999.[17] Investigators found that asthma patients in the experimental group showed significant improvements in lung function (increase of FEV_1 from 63.9 percent at baseline to 76.3 percent at the four-month follow-up), whereas control group patients showed no change. Similarly, rheumatoid arthritis patients in the experimental group showed a significant reduction of 28 percent in overall disease severity at the four-month follow-up, whereas control group patients did not change. Combining all 107 patients, 47.1 percent of experimental patients had clinically relevant improvement, whereas only 24.3 percent of control patients had improvement.

A suggestion to a patient by a healthcare provider regarding the value of journaling may open up a new avenue for coping and perhaps even improvement in the disease.

REFLECTIONS

- In what ways do you assist patients with chronic illnesses to cope with their situation?
- What is your experience with the use of and power of prayer in the lives of those with chronic illnesses?
- Have you ever taught a patient to use the "Faith Factor" with the Relaxation Response technique? If so, what was the result?
- Have you ever used music or books as part of your care of patients? What happened as a result of using these interventions?
- Have you ever encouraged patients to use journaling? If so, what happened?

✶ Do you journal? Consider starting a journal. Write down the most significant experience of your day and reflect on why it was significant.

One of our participants, Brenda Thornton, a medical homecare nurse, remembers the four years she spent caring for Floyd, a patient who suffered from chronic illness and pain.

The first time I met him, he had a below-the-knee amputation; he smoked constantly, using the butt of one cigarette to light the next one; he had a huge sacral decubitus; his circulation was terrible; and he was angry and verbally abusive. To add to all this, he was racist, and I am black. He had already refused care from many other nurses, most of them white. I wasn't confident that I stood a chance with Floyd. During our first visit, I calmly told him what I was going to do and remained nonreactive to his slurs and side comments. When I was finished with his dressing change, I sat and talked to him. I shared that although he seemed to dislike blacks, I was convinced that God loves all of us and sees the inside of us, not the color of our skin.

I visited Floyd twice a day, seven days a week. I remained calm and nonjudgmental toward him. Even though it took a long time for him to soften in his outward behavior, I was the only nurse he would allow to provide the twice-a-day care. If I were off for some reason, he would let another nurse come in only once a day, and was rude and nasty to whomever came in my place.

There was also a black home health aide who worked with Floyd. This young man was incredibly kind and really went above and beyond the call of duty when caring for Floyd. He helped Floyd get out of bed, he bought him cigarettes and other things to brighten Floyd's day. He really showed him love. Then one day Floyd was in a particularly ugly mood and called this young man the N-word. The aide was hurt and angry and didn't want to ever go back to care for Floyd.

I spoke to the aide about the fact that Floyd was angry, but not at the aide. Floyd was angry at himself, at God, and at the world. Then I went to see Floyd, and we had a heart-to-heart talk. I told him that what he had done to the aide was unacceptable, that it was hurtful and hateful behavior that not only impacted on the aide but on me as well, since I am black. I talked to him about the fact that he was receiving the love of God through us even though he acted in an unloving way and that I had reached the end of my rope and would no longer accept this behavior.

Well, miracles never cease! Floyd apologized to the aide and to me. He softened and became more open. I never preached to him—that would have been inappropriate—but we talked a lot about God. His medical condition worsened. His other leg was amputated, first below the knee and then above the knee. By the time he died, only small stumps of his legs remained. The doctors tried everything to heal the sacral decubitus, but Floyd was unable to be compliant with his part of the treatment, like staying off his back. He finally succumbed to sepsis, but he was a different man than the angry person I had met four years before. He was at peace with himself and with God.

REFLECTIONS

- As you read Brenda's story of Floyd, can you describe the spiritual interventions that she provided? What about the home health aide?
- What do you think Floyd hoped for? In what was his hope centered?
- How was trust developed between Brenda and Floyd?
- Why do you think that Floyd was so angry? How would you have responded to Floyd? Could you have continued to provide care to him while he continued his abusive behavior and racist talk?
- Referring to chapter 5, describe how Brenda provided ministries of presence, action, and word.

Chronic illness is a major focus for most healthcare providers. Heart disease, diabetes, and asthma are now the leading causes of chronic illness in the United States today. The Medicare and Medicaid programs currently spend $84 billion annually on five major chronic conditions, specifically diabetes (17 million people), heart disease (13 million people with coronary artery disease and 50 million with hypertension), depression, cancer, and arthritis.[18] A recent international health study, conducted by the World Health Organization and the World Bank in conjunction with Harvard Medical School, concluded that the largest health problems of the next quarter-century will be chronic conditions, especially those that affect the elderly.[19] By the year 2020, they predict that lung disease related to smoking will be the world's greatest killer. Furthermore, mental illness—led by depressive disorders—will be the second-most-disabling condition after heart disease.

We are concerned with providing comfort, limiting disability, providing relief from pain, controlling the illness, maintaining independence, and facilitating quality of life. Just as important, however, is the need to be concerned and to take action regarding the spiritual aspects of chronic illness. There is so much we can do if we are willing to extend our practices to include the spiritual.

In the next chapter, we continue to examine the role of spirituality in specific patient situations such as the dying patient, the patient with AIDS, and the patient facing surgery; the care of sick children; and meeting the needs of caregivers.

[7]

Giving Spiritual Care
The Dying Patient

> *For everything its season, and for everything*
> *under heaven its time:*
> *a time to be born and a time to die,*
> *a time to plant and a time to uproot,*
> *a time to kill and a time to heal,*
> *a time to pull down and a time to build up,*
> *a time for mourning and a time for dancing,*
> *a time for silence and a time for speech.*
> —*Ecclesiastes 3:1–7*

As an oncology nurse, Miriam Jacik had many occasions to see and experience patients or their family members grappling with the meaning of illness, suffering, and death.

Spiritual ministry extends to the care of the terminally ill and dying persons. When faced with the proximity of death, be it days, weeks, or months from the present time, a person is led to look at the deeper meaning of the experiences that life brings. There is a prioritizing of those things that are found to be an inher-

TABLE 4. Needs of Dying Persons Viewed from a
Whole-Person Perspective

Biological	Emotional	Social	Spiritual
Adequate treat- ment and care	Hope Respect	Presence of loved ones	Forgiveness— reconciliation
Caring health providers	Control Honesty/open	Time to share with spouse/	Prayer—religious services
Prudent medical management	communication	children Permission to die	Spiritual assistance at death
Comfort		Finished business	Peace

Taken from M. Jacik, "Spiritual Care of the Dying Adult," 266.

ently valuable part of one's existence. The ministering person, if aware, is privi-
leged to be a part of that process and discovers, with the person who is approach-
ing her or his death, that family and friends, as well as personal beliefs and val-
ues, are truly treasured components of the person's life. These far outweigh in
importance all the material, financial, educational, and professional successes
achieved in a lifetime.

Walking in gratitude with one who has made such a discovery is a blessed
experience! The ministering person supports and affirms as the dying person
strives to cherish every moment that can be spent with those who are held dear.
The ministering person encourages clinging to those values and beliefs that have
brought meaning in life, so that these same values and beliefs may bring mean-
ing in death.

Patients who are facing death experience physical, emotional, social,
and spiritual needs. Healthcare providers who are privileged to work
with the dying must be sensitive to the whole range of needs. Table 4
presents the needs of the dying from a whole-person perspective.

Let's take a closer look at the spiritual needs of the dying person,
which include forgiveness and reconciliation, prayer and religious services, spiritual assistance at death, and a sense of peace.

FORGIVENESS AND RECONCILIATION

Dying persons often approach death overwhelmed or troubled by the fact that in certain relationships they have never granted or received forgiveness. Perhaps they were hurt or offended by insensitive or selfish things that were said or done to them. Perhaps they experienced rejection from significant others in their lives. Perhaps they can't even remember the reason for the separation. But they know for sure that the result of the offense was division, silence, bitterness, and deep-seated pain. They know there has never been reconciliation or a mending of broken ties, and they are uneasy going to their death with unsettled issues.[1] Sometimes patients seek forgiveness and reconciliation from loved ones or friends; other times patients seek forgiveness from their God.

In a study with terminal patients, Kaldjian and colleagues underscored the importance of spiritual concerns, including the issue of forgiveness.[2] The study group consisted of mostly African-American Christian HIV-positive patients. Ninety patients were asked their views about God, forgiveness, their feelings about the disease, their resuscitation status, fear of death, use of prayer and Scripture, and whether they possessed a living will.

Overwhelmingly (98 percent), this group expressed belief in God and God's forgiveness (81 percent). HIV disease was considered a form of punishment by 26 percent of the respondents; 17 percent believed that punishment came from God; 44 percent expressed guilt about their HIV status. Those who expressed guilt about their HIV status or who believed that disease was a punishment from God were more likely to express fear about death. Those who read the Bible daily, weekly, or monthly and those who considered God an integral part of the meaning of their lives were less likely to fear death. Those who prayed daily were 7.9 times as likely to possess a living will; those who believed in God's forgiveness were more likely to participate in discussions of resuscitation.

In a national Gallup survey that asked about the concerns expressed by respondents regarding dying, forgiveness was ranked as the most significant concern. In fact, the top-rated spiritual concerns were, in this order, "not being forgiven by God" (56 percent of respondents), "not reconciling with others" (56 percent), "dying when removed or cut off from God" (51 percent), and "not being forgiven by someone for a wrongdoing" (49 percent).[3] Clearly, forgiveness weighs heavily on the hearts of those who are dying.

Catherine Lick, a parish nurse, recounts the story of a seventy-five-year-old woman who was dealing with the issue of forgiveness as she prepared for her own death.

Pat was suffering from cancer as well as the results of a stroke. The cancer affected the mobility of her right arm; the stroke affected the mobility of her left arm. She was very disabled and ready to die. When I visited her, she talked about how difficult her marriage had been. Her husband had been openly involved in extra-marital affairs and he was dictatorial and controlling. She felt she should forgive him but felt nothing but disdain.

Over many visits we prayed together. I used touch, presence, listening, and Scripture. On one visit she asked me to pray with her about this issue of forgiveness. She believed she should forgive but was unable to do so. I shared with her that I believed that the Spirit of God is able to help us forgive others when we lack the ability to do so on our own. I told her the story of Corrie Ten Boom, who was asked for forgiveness by one of the guards who had helped to imprison her and her family during World War II. At first Corrie Ten Boom was repulsed by the guard's request; she could not forgive him. But then she felt the Spirit of God move her to reach out her hand to the guard in forgiveness.

Pat asked that we pray together that the Lord would help her forgive. On another visit, Pat asked me if it was okay for her to pray for the Lord to take her. I shared with her that we are just sojourners on this earth, and a desire to return to God is proper.

What are the interventions available to healthcare providers who face a patient's concerns about forgiveness? What can we do to assist in the process of forgiveness? We can't force anyone to forgive another person. It is a personal choice to forgive or not. In fact, some would argue that it is God's intervention that allows us to forgive. Through attentive listening and the ministry of our presence, however, we may learn that the patient carries deep pain regarding a broken relationship. We can

The role of the healthcare professional in facilitating forgiveness is to listen to the patient's story, to validate the pain, to ask questions and clarify the issues, to inquire about the patient's desire to do something about the broken relationship, and to ask whether we can be of any assistance in the process.

𝔞

Prayer provides support and comfort to the dying person. When you offer to pray with someone who is struggling to do so because of pain and weakness, you bridge the gap between the patient and God.

comment on what we see and hear. We can empathize with the pain the patient is expressing in regard to this relationship. We can ask if there is something that the patient would like to do about the relationship. We can ask how the patient would like to go about mending the relationship. Lastly, we can ask if there is something we can do to assist the patient. Sometimes just putting feelings into words encourages the other person to explore issues in a different way. We can't force forgiveness, but we can certainly facilitate it.

PRAYER AND RELIGIOUS SERVICES

Offering to pray with a dying person can be a source of comfort and strength. In the face of impending death, we are frequently at a loss for words. We want to say something that will make it all better, that will take away pain and will change the outcome. We are powerless to do any of these things. We can, however, put voice to the patient's feelings and offer those concerns to God.

In *The Journey to Peace*, a book written by Cardinal Joseph Bernardin during the final months of his life as he struggled in the last stages of pancreatic cancer, the cardinal talked about the importance of having a praying network that could provide support to a person facing death. He shared how difficult it was for him to pray even though he had been a man of deep prayer most of his life. He also commented on how important it was to be prayed for; the support and love that emanate from prayer is like scaffolding that holds up the dying when personal resources are depleted.[4]

Jacik suggests that offers to pray with the patient are most helpful when they are made weeks and days before death. Waiting until the patient is slipping in and out of consciousness is not particularly beneficial to the patient, even though it may be very helpful to the family gathered at the patient's bedside.[5]

Religious services, such as the reception of the sacraments, anointing with oil, or receiving a blessing of departure are very meaningful to patients and their families. According to Koenig, these "religious practices facilitate coping and are used to regulate emotion during times of illness, change and circumstances that are out of patients' personal control."[6] These services can be provided by either the chaplain or the pastoral care department, or by clergy from the patient's faith community. Physician Herman Brecher remembers a situation where he actually performed a necessary religious service: "I was taking care of a newborn that was dying, and there was no priest available. With the assistance of the nurse, I baptized the child prior to death. This was very important to the mother, and she was most appreciative."

SPIRITUAL ASSISTANCE AT DEATH

In addition to having family and members of one's faith tradition at the deathbed, the presence of a healthcare provider who is intermittently at the bedside and remains readily available during the long hours of the dying process provides valuable spiritual assistance. Hospice provides this care to patients who choose to die at home. This action says to the patient and family that the patient will be accompanied through the dying process. Physical presence is a powerful spiritual intervention and an invaluable gift that can be offered to dying persons and their families. "One Hour and Twelve Minutes" is a story of presence.

ONE HOUR AND TWELVE MINUTES

I began working in healthcare in September of 1984. Having been raised by parents who were both nurses, I was not surprised that my own career path led me to a profession in healthcare. I had recently graduated from seminary, and chose to enter a year of intense healthcare-based pastoral training known as clinical pastoral education. Though I interviewed at several centers, I knew from the start that I wanted to train at Baylor University Medical Center in Dallas, Texas. Baylor was located near the downtown area of Dallas and provided all the challenges for which

I hoped. It included a major trauma center, a thriving transplant program, a large oncology practice, and much more. I could hardly wait to be a part of such an exciting place. I was thrilled when I was accepted into the pastoral care program.

Early in the orientation week, we were given our floor assignments for the next year. My dream came true as I read "Emergency Department" next to my name. To my surprise, however, the letters "L&D" also appeared. I assumed most of my education would come from my experiences in the emergency and trauma areas. I could not have been more mistaken.

It was a Thursday evening, and I was the chaplain for the entire hospital. The other chaplains had left for home, and I prepared to respond to whatever the evening had in store. I had been training for all of two months. My pager alerted me around 8 PM that I was needed in Labor and Delivery. When I arrived, the charge nurse told me that a young family had requested to see a chaplain. They had been admitted earlier in the day, fearing that their baby was about to be born after only twenty-eight weeks of gestation. Their worst fears were realized, and the baby was born shortly after I had been called. After extensive emergency care, the medical team offered no hope for the baby's survival. I was led into the room where the twenty-two-year-old dad and the twenty-year-old mom were holding their firstborn, a baby girl named Cassie Leigh. On either side of the bed stood the grandparents, gathered to care for their own children, who were experiencing the most difficult day anyone could imagine. Everyone in the room had tears rolling down their cheeks.

At twenty-five years old, I was still quite naïve about life and death, and I had no clue how I might be of comfort to this grieving family. Initially, I stood inside the door, apprehensive about what to say or do. Somehow, though, I managed to introduce myself and tell them that I was there to offer support. With a shaky voice and a trembling hand, the young dad introduced me to his new baby daughter. Cassie had not only been born prematurely, but she also had severe internal anomalies. Mom and Dad recounted the events of the day, carefully including each detail they held precious. Words are insufficient to relate the emotions of their story. Alternating between the dreams of a healthy daughter and the painful reality they now faced, they were somehow about to appreciate that, if only for a brief moment, Cassie was with them.

Somewhere in our conversation, Cassie's mom asked me if I wanted to hold Cassie. I took her and ever so gently held her. Having grown up with no younger siblings and quite afraid of babies, this was a new experience for me! I then handed her to a grandparent. For the next few minutes we all took turns holding Cassie. Periodically the nurse came back to check on everyone and to listen to Cassie's heart. At one point she told us that Cassie would not survive much longer.

With everyone gathered around, I held Cassie and said a prayer, acknowledging that she had affected me in a way for which I was not prepared. Placing her back in her mother's arms, I stood expectantly and watched this little baby touch us all. A few moments later the doctor entered, listened to Cassie's heart, and told us she had died. Though this news was expected, everyone was devastated.

I remained with the family for a while longer, wishing that in seminary I had been given the magical words that would make everything better. No such words exist. Instead we all grieved and tried to console each other. As I was about to leave, I promised to pray for them and offered to help in any way I could. Turning toward the door, I was stopped by Cassie's mom. With a tired and trembling voice she spoke these words, words I will never forget: "Jeff, you are the only minister who Cassie ever knew, and you are the only minister who ever knew Cassie. It would mean so much to us if you would preach her funeral."

My mind tried to say no, but my heart and my mouth overruled my mind and said yes. What could I possibly say at the funeral? As a young naïve minister, I knew I was in over my head. During the next three days, I pondered what philosophical or theological truths might bring comfort to this family. Terrified, I simply told everyone who gathered on that cool Monday afternoon that Cassie Leigh had touched us all, and that life could never be measured in terms of days, weeks, or years but rather by its impact. The lesson she had taught me was that we all impact the lives of those around us, particularly those whom we love, and we have the opportunity to do so in a positive way. While she could not use words, Cassie had given us all a new understanding of what it means to love and be loved.

The medical record reflected that Cassie lived one hour and twelve minutes.

But for me, she still lives. She reminds me that each life is precious and that the care we give others in healthcare is special. It is a sacred privilege to be invited to journey with people in times of sadness or celebration. We should not take these encounters for granted, but rather be open to what we might experience. While I hope I gave care to this family, I am positive they gave care to me.

During the rest of that year, I had many of the experiences I had anticipated. I worked with trauma victims, visited the transplant patients, and even published a paper on bone marrow transplants. However, none of the countless hours spent on those experiences touched me as much as that one hour and twelve minutes.

—W. Jeffrey Flowers

Sandra Brown, a family nurse practitioner, shares two stories of the use of music to provide spiritual assistance.

I was with the family and patient, and basically we were waiting for him to die. He was too weak to do anything—even moving in bed and talking were too much of an effort. He just lay quietly, breathing very slowly and with some difficulty. Occasionally he would open his eyes and look at everyone in the room. His family shared that he had loved to sing in church, so another nurse and I, who were taking care of him, gathered around his bed and began to sing his favorite hymns. He opened his eyes and actually began to sing!

On another occasion, Sandy was present when a family was saying good-bye to a beloved daughter. "The family had reached a point where they were finally ready to release their daughter to God. This had been a terribly difficult journey for them. We held hands around the bed and sang songs of faith as she took her last breath. It was a very sad moment, but I felt so privileged to be present to them and to be able to participate in this sending off of this young woman to God."

Dr. Daniel Ober, the medical director of a hospice program, frequently counsels "patients and families who are confronting unbelievable suffering. I offer them spiritual comfort, and many times I am able to draw from my own experiences to assist them in finding their own answers."

Dr. Sandra Jamison, a retired nurse, recounts a story of providing spiritual care to an elderly woman who belonged to Dr. Jamison's church.

This lady was dying of cancer. She wanted to remain in her home but didn't have a caregiver. Her daughter lived in a foreign country and was unable to immediately come home to care for her mother. I offered to organize the care, and I stayed with her every night. One of the most precious times I had with her occurred one evening when she was in a lot of pain and very restless. She asked me to read the Bible to her, which I did. After reading a passage, I would ask her if there were other passages that she would like me to read, and she made some suggestions. I also sang hymns while I sat with her. The Scripture reading and the hymns produced a visible calm in her.

Sometimes dying patients and families minister to us. We are touched by the courage they display and the peace that they feel as they prepare for the inevitable. Such is the case in this story from Karen McCauley, a homecare nurse.

I will never forget this one patient and his wife. I saw them for over a year, and I believe they ministered to me. My patient required Foley catheter care as a result of benign prostrate hypertrophy. I had been seeing him for a while when he started having bloody urine and was taken to the hospital, where he was diagnosed with cancer. The primary site of the tumor was unknown. After he received the diagnosis, he deteriorated rapidly. He was in extreme pain, and I continued to work closely with the patient and his family for pain management.

We talked about a lot of things, including God and the patient's expected dying. He was more accepting and at peace than I was. His pain continued to intensify, and none of the medications were working. Finally it was clear that his dying was imminent, and he was in such awful pain. I was so upset with myself for not being able to help him that the last day I saw him alive I actually broke down and cried. I apologized to him and his wife, and they comforted me and reassured me that I had done a good job. Can you imagine, the patient was facing his own death and still able to reach out to me!

Evelyn Yapp, a psychiatric nurse, offers another story of how a dying patient touched her deeply.

Last year I lost a patient to liver cirrhosis after years of drug abuse. She gave me the opportunity to learn how it is to suffer and cope with that suffering through faith. But what I witnessed with her and her friends was that everyone was touched and changed by her dying. To be honest, I was surprised by what I saw. I knew this woman as a person who received psychotherapy from me. Yet as she approached her death, she transcended all of those issues that had burdened her for so long. She changed into a spiritual being as she moved from this life to the next. It was an amazing experience for me and gave me such a sense of awe for the power of God to transform. This experience made me more aware of the transitory nature of what we do but also the spiritual significance of what we do. I am looking at everything in my life—my relationships with family, friends, and work associates—and reevaluating these in terms of their spiritual significance and meaning.

REFLECTIONS

- What is your experience in providing care to dying persons? What spiritual interventions have you used in that care?
- Can you think of a patient where the need for forgiveness and reconciliation was apparent to you? How did you handle this?
- How have you facilitated religious services? What is your level of participation if the patient and family request a religious service at the bedside?
- What is your experience praying with or for a dying patient? How did you pray?

SPIRITUAL NEEDS OF GRIEVING CAREGIVERS AND FAMILIES

It is not just dying persons that we must consider. Sometimes we encounter families who are anticipating grief. Their loved one has received a terminal diagnosis, and they are confronted with the incomprehensible—the loss of their beloved.

"The Diagnosis" provides a glimpse into that initial grief, as we hear Mary's reaction to her husband's diagnosis.

THE DIAGNOSIS

I sat next to Paul as the doctor gave us the diagnosis of lung cancer. I felt as if I were watching from afar—disconnected yet fully aware of all that was going on. I heard the words, and I could see how uncomfortable the doctor was in the telling. I found myself wondering, "This should be easier for him to say; he probably does it all the time." I heard him describe Paul's treatment options, and I began to weigh the pros and cons in my mind. I heard him say something about Paul and me having at least one more good year. I was quite objective and rational. Three days later while cleaning up the kitchen, I broke down and began to cry. I sobbed for a long time. The realization that my husband of forty years was going to die hit me with the power of a raging storm. I was flooded with thoughts of being alone, of not having him to share my life with. I felt afraid. I felt angry, but at whom? At Paul? At the cancer? At God? I didn't know. I wanted to run away from the reality as if I could somehow change it. I found myself praying—begging God for a miracle. "Dear Lord, please let this be a mistake, a horrible mistake. Let my Paul live." Somehow I knew that this was not a mistake, that I was embarking on the most difficult journey of my life, and I desperately needed God to walk alongside of me.[7]

The spiritual issues inherent in the role of grieving caregiver include:

- The experience of intense pain associated with grieving
- The need to know that there is a loving and sustaining God in the midst of the pain
- The desire to emulate God's love, patience, and faithfulness as the caregiving role is fulfilled
- The need to have answers to the ultimate question of why
- The need to feel connected to a greater and more powerful Being who is able to make sense out of pain and death
- The need for forgiveness when expectations and behaviors are incongruent

The continuation of Mary's story, "Spiritual Pain," illustrates these needs.

SPIRITUAL PAIN

Some days I prayed for Paul's healing even though I knew deep in my heart that he would not be healed. Other times I prayed for myself—that God would take away my pain. There were times it was so intense that I could barely function; I prayed that He would give me the love, strength, patience, and fortitude to be there for Paul whenever he needed me. I felt inadequate to the task. There were other days that I couldn't pray—I was just too tired; I had given too much; I felt spent and unable to put into words what I needed. At other times I relied on God to be there for me and understand what seemed incomprehensible to me. The one question that I asked God over and over again was, Why? Why Paul? Why me? Why us?

As Paul got weaker, there were days when I felt angry at him that he couldn't do more. I was so tired and weary. I was afraid of his death; yet there were times when I longed for release from the burden of constant care. I could barely tolerate the pain of such thoughts. I begged God to forgive me for such thoughts, and I prayed He would help me forgive myself. [8]

What can we do to assist a caregiver who is experiencing anticipatory grieving? First of all, we can acknowledge that the caregiving journey is a difficult one; we can offer our presence and our desire to listen; we can suggest resources that might lighten the burden of caregiving; we can offer to support the caregiver and the patient with prayer. Although it is important to respect the religious beliefs of caregivers and patients, spiritual care is not tied to a particular religion or faith tradition. Rather, it is tied to transcendent values of love, faithfulness, generosity, and selflessness, which are inherent to many faith traditions. In addition, spiritual care is intimately linked with the desire to understand the meaning and purpose of life itself; to make sense out of pain and suffering; to believe that there is a reason for everything, most importantly those things that cause anguish and heartache; and to feel connected to God (however God is defined) and to others.

The last part of Mary's story, "Spiritual Care," illustrates how Mary's needs were met.

SPIRITUAL CARE

There were days when I felt all alone. I needed to talk, but Paul was not up to talking; he was too weak, and he needed to rest. Sometimes I felt surrounded by death and longed for a new life and a sense of rebirth. Yet overall I felt sustained. Friends and family reached out to me in wonderful ways. One day I walked into my kitchen and found my whole dinner sitting on my kitchen table. Another day my sister stopped by after work carrying a bunch of fresh spring flowers. She thought my spirit needed some lifting. She was right! And the prayer support— how could I have managed without it? I always knew that when I was unable to pray, others were praying for me. So many people offered a listening ear and allowed me to vent my pain, frustrations, and fears. I remember several weekends when my friends came to our house and relieved me of my caregiving responsibilities so I could get away to do whatever I wanted. Those were real gifts to both Paul and me; they were answers to prayer that I will treasure forever. Without this support, I am not sure that I could have been there for Paul.[9]

A family whose loved one has died has similar needs for prayer and spiritual assistance. All too often, however, grieving families are forgotten once their loved one is buried. The connections the family developed with caring health professionals are cut off, and they must traverse the course of grieving alone. Support groups for grieving families are not as available as they should be. Families would benefit from continued contact with the healthcare providers who stood by them while they waited for their loved ones to die. Periodic telephone calls to offer support and encouragement provide families with the message that they are not forgotten. Calls on special occasions such as birthdays, holidays, and anniversaries are particularly useful, because losses are more acutely felt on these occasions.[10]

A research study conducted by Dr. Michael King and colleagues at the Royal Free and University College Medical School in London found that people with strong spiritual beliefs may recover from the death of a close relative or friend more quickly than people who lack such beliefs.[11]

The study involved monitoring the grieving process among 129 relatives and close friends of patients with terminal illnesses. Forty-three percent of the study group reported having strong religious beliefs, 41 percent said they had "low religious beliefs," and 16 percent said they had no religious beliefs.

Among the 95 people who participated in follow-up studies, the people with strong religious beliefs showed the most positive recovery from bereavement, reporting progressively less grief at one-, nine-, and fourteen-month follow-up sessions. Those who reported low religious beliefs reported little change in their grief until after the nine-month interval passed, after which they experienced rapid recovery. Those who reported no religious beliefs reported a brief improvement between the one- and nine-month follow-ups, but they experienced an intense sensation of grief that was still evident at the fourteen-month follow-up. The researchers speculated that people with spiritual beliefs fared better than others because many of them take a longer or different view of life and what it means, and consider life after death.

Miriam Jacik, a nurse as well as a pastoral counselor, currently conducts a bereavement support group at her church. She reflects on this experience:

At the present time while working as a grief counselor I am able to reach out to the needs of grieving persons. These needs are emotional, spiritual, and relational. They are deep and there is much pain. Once again there is anger at God who would allow someone to die, leaving behind families who need them. With some resolution of that anger there is a turning to God, religion, and prayer to obtain the strength to complete the grief process. It calls me to draw upon the spirituality and religious beliefs that I hold sacred. It allows me to reach out in compassion and caring to others, helping them to fathom the mysteries of life and death.[12]

Rodger Murchison shares his experiences of working with the bereaved:

I was conducting a grief workshop at my church. I feel a com- Grieving families
mitment to do this, since there is such a link between health have similar needs
problems and unresolved grief. Tom, whose wife died two years for spiritual assis-
ago, wanted to be more social. He felt ready to get involved in tance, prayer, and
life again. Yet he felt guilty doing so. He believed his wife was participation in
watching over him with disapproval. I suggested that he write religious services.
a letter to his wife and take it to her grave and read it. In the Their needs continue
letter I suggested that he ask his wife to release him in all long after their loved
ways. Tom followed through with this and reported that he felt one has died.
relieved and free from the guilt that had been nagging him.

I remember another situation where I intervened, involving Ruth, whose husband of sixty years had passed away about a year ago. Ruth continued to visit her husband's grave at least twice a week and spent the entire visit crying. Her grief was immobilizing her. I suggested that she needed to relocate her husband. I told her that her husband was not present in the grave, but rather he was in heaven and in a better place. My suggestion to her was that if she wasn't able to let him die, he wouldn't allow her to live. Ruth was able to psychologically relocate her husband and move on.

REFLECTIONS

- What are your personal experiences with loss? How did you handle your grief? What actions provided by others were helpful to you?
- What were your spiritual needs during your grief period?
- Is there anything you can do to make sure that those who are grieving are not "forgotten" by the healthcare system?
- Have you worked with families or individual caregivers who were dealing with anticipatory grief? In what ways were you able to assist them?
- In your personal life, have you experienced anticipatory grief? What were your spiritual needs, and how were they met?

As healthcare providers, we have a role in providing spiritual care to those who are dying, to those who are caring for the dying, and to those who grieve for their deceased loved one. We can't change the outcome, but we can provide our presence, our listening ear, and our willingness to accompany them as they walk this path. We might be able to facilitate forgiveness, to provide prayer support, and to arrange for deeply desired religious services that help the patient and family bear up under incredible sorrow.

Let's continue our examination of spiritual care. In chapter 8, we examine other patient situations, such as caring for the patient with AIDS, the psychiatric patient, the surgical patient, and the patient with dementia.

[8]

Spiritual Care for Special Populations

To be a patient is to be one who is patient, one who endures. To be a patient is to be one who suffers not only in the sense of allowing pain, of acknowledging and incorporating it as a true thing that is actually happening and that must be dealt with as such. The power of acknowledgment and incorporation—the power to exercise the freedom to establish an identity and maintain integrity—is the power available to and essential for the suffering ones we wish to serve. It is the power that our recognition of their suffering can evoke and enhance.

—Margaret E. Mohrmann, *Medicine as Ministry*

The introductory quotation reinforces a key component of spiritual care: to first recognize that even though we may not be able to remove the suffering of our patients, we are called upon to give witness and affirmation to their suffering. This aspect of spiritual care is enough to shore up the patient's sense of self and contributes to the patient's endurance—the ability, as Mohrmann puts it, "that looks at suffering square in the face, sees it for what it is, and then decides what is to be done about it. It is in this process of clear vision, open acknowledgment, and careful decision that endurance produces character, the sort of character that is full of hope that neither suffering nor anything else will separate the sufferer from God."[1]

This chapter examines spiritual care provided to people who endure —the patient with AIDS, the psychiatric patient, and the dementia patient, as well as the caregivers of these patients; children with chronic illnesses and their parents; and the surgical patient.

AIDS PATIENTS

Today AIDS is viewed from the perspective of a chronic illness and as such has spiritual issues similar to other chronic illnesses. (See chapter 6 for more discussion of chronic illnesses and spirituality.) There are some characteristics of AIDS, however, that set it apart from other chronic diseases like diabetes, congestive heart failure, or chronic obstructive pulmonary disease. AIDS is transmissible and stigmatizing.[2] It brands its victims as being either homosexual or drug users. There are other means by which the disease is transmitted (through blood transfusions; from infected mother to newborn; and via heterosexual contact, as is the case with 90 percent of AIDS cases in Africa), but, generally speaking, AIDS is associated with lifestyle issues that make many in society uncomfortable.

The disease is frequently approached from a moralistic perspective. Kayal discusses what happens when the etiology of a disease is framed in moral language, and the illness in question affects individuals who have been "religiously stigmatized and legally proscribed minorities."[3] The afflicted are blamed for their illness, and this has certainly taken place with AIDS. Consequently, there are many spiritual issues associated with the disease. Those who are diagnosed with AIDS may experience rejection not only from family and friends but also from their faith community, leaving them isolated and feeling cut off from God. There are some in society who contend that AIDS is a just punishment for homosexual behavior and clearly believe that the disease is God's punishment. Claiming the authority of God increases the accuser's credibility as well as the social alienation felt by the person with AIDS (PWA).

AIDS challenges Americans to examine persistent attitudes about the ministrations of comfort and compassion, acceptance of individual differences, and society's responsibility to deal with the suffering of its young. These are not challenges to be addressed easily or without pain, and AIDS has certainly brought them into sharp focus.

In her book *AIDS: The Ultimate Challenge*, Elisabeth Kübler-Ross speaks to the challenge facing our country in the care of PWAs: "Since we can no longer deny that AIDS is a life threatening illness that will eventually involve millions of people and decimate large portions of our human population, it is our choice to grow and learn from it, to either help people with this dread disease or abandon them. It is our choice to live up to this ultimate challenge or to perish."[4]

> Those who are diagnosed with AIDS may experience rejection not only from family and friends but also from their faith community, leaving them isolated and feeling cut off from God.

What happens to the PWA who is caught up in this societal struggle? Sometimes the PWA is left to deal with the illness in isolation. The victim of societal homophobia—an irrational fear, intolerance, and dread on the part of heterosexual people to be in close proximity to any person believed to be homosexual—the PWA is rejected, condemned, and ostracized. Murphy quotes a young homosexual who, when a counselor was attempting to assure the young man of God's love, said, "How can God love me? I am one of his mistakes."[5]

The PWA who is faced with death must contemplate many spiritual issues.

Self-identity—characterized by questions such as, Who am I now? Am I still the same person even though my body fails me daily? Does anyone still love me for who I am?

Meaning of life—characterized by questions such as, Is there some value to my suffering and loss? Has my life been important?

Adversity—characterized by questions such as, Is life always so cruel? Can there be anything worse than an unfair death?

Fate—characterized by questions such as, Why has this happened to me? Why must I be deprived of the life I love?

Stigma—characterized by questions such as, Is this a punishment for being gay—for being who I am?

Relationships—characterized by fears such as, Will my lover leave me? Will my friends and family reject and abandon me?

Productivity—characterized by concerns such as, I've lost my job. I feel so weak, and I'm fatigued doing the slightest tasks. Am I of any use to anyone?

Heritage—characterized by concerns such as, What can I leave behind? How will people remember me?[6]

Coming to grips with these spiritual issues is frequently complicated by unresolved conflicts over life choices, such as IV drug use or guilt over sexual activities that exposed the person to the HIV virus. Further complicating this spiritual quest is low self-esteem, social isolation and alienation, and public discrimination and condemnation.

Homecare nurse Florie Miranda provided intravenous infusion care to young men with AIDS. Florie's story illustrates the spiritual struggle that confronts the PWA.

I did this work in the early 1990s, and societal attitudes about homosexuality and AIDS have changed a bit since then. I remember one young man who was dying with AIDS. His mother and father were of Italian descent and had come to the United States from the "old country." Their son had moved away from home and relocated to the West Coast. He had prospered in business, had a full social life, and was able to live openly as a homosexual. However, when he became ill, he returned home to the East Coast and back to his parents' home.

He did not return home to loving acceptance. His parents were ashamed, angry, and certainly at times living in denial. They cared for him begrudgingly and refused to allow any of his gay friends to visit him. They told all their family and friends that their son was dying of cancer; they absolutely refused to openly acknowledge that he was gay and that he was dying of AIDS.

I tried to talk to them. On one occasion I sat at the dining room table with his mom and dad and attempted to discuss how difficult this situation was for their son. The father banged his fist on the table, got up, and walked away from me. His mother said over and over again, "I'm sorry—we just can't talk about this." It was clear that I was this young man's sole support—emotionally and spiritually.

As he received the intravenous infusions, I had a lot of time to spend with him. We talked about his life, his illness, his significant other, his desires for the rest of his life and for his death. We talked about God. We talked about forgiveness. I listened to him. We laughed together and we cried together. I felt it was important in this last stage of his life that he felt accepted and loved—I believe that he felt that.

Considering these spiritual issues, the question is, what is the health-care provider's role in responding to spirituality in the patient with AIDS? Before addressing that question, it is incumbent that we examine our own attitudes toward homosexuality and the disease of AIDS. If self-examination reveals that we harbor judgment and condemnation toward such patients, then we have no place in their care. On the other hand, if we are able to see the suffering of this person and respond with the ability to listen, to be present, to offer compassion and concern, then we are able to render spiritual care.

REFLECTIONS

- Have you provided care to AIDS patients?
- What were the spiritual needs of those patients?
- In what ways were you able to meet those needs?
- Reread Florie's story. What are the spiritual issues of the young man that Florie describes?
- If a patient with AIDS described rejection from a faith community and was angry at God, how would you respond to this patient's spiritual need?

PSYCHIATRIC PATIENTS

Another group of patients who have significant spiritual needs are those with psychiatric illnesses. Some feel angry with God for allowing them to suffer with disorders that affect every aspect of their lives. Some patients have issues of forgiveness to address, such as when friends and family have responded to the patient with rejection and hurtful comments and attitudes just because the patient suffers with a psychiatric illness. Other patients may need to seek forgiveness because of hurt they have caused to others during a psychiatric episode. Many patients rely on God as their source of love and support and display a deep, abiding faith despite the circumstances of their illnesses.

The challenge in meeting these spiritual needs in the psychiatric patient occurs with respecting boundary issues. Boundary issues deal with defining the respective roles of caregiver versus patient and with defining the limits of one's own identity. It is not uncommon in psychiatric illnesses for patients to have "loose boundaries," especially in the presence of a psychotic or personality disorder. Patients may experience difficulty knowing where their beliefs stop and those of the healthcare professional begin.

This places the patient in a vulnerable position of perhaps being unfairly influenced by someone of strong and imposing beliefs. In meeting the spiritual needs of psychiatric patients, it is imperative that we are continually aware and respectful of boundary issues, and never impose our spiritual beliefs on the patient. With this caveat in mind, it is important that healthcare professionals consider the spiritual needs of patients and respond to these needs through the use of presence and caring actions and words.

There is abundant research demonstrating the positive relationship between religion and measures of well-being, including marital status, health, activities, social support, optimism, hope, purpose and meaning in life, and internal locus of control.[7] During the twentieth century, there were at least 724 quantitative studies that examined these relationships. Nearly 500 (66 percent) found a statistically significant relationship between religious involvement and better mental health.[8] This is especially true for studies looking at positive emotions—well-being, hope, optimism—where nearly 80 percent find significant associations with religious faith and practice. These studies, however, do not reflect the many persons with mental illness whose religious faith has deepened as a result of their suffering, and yet they continue to struggle—their heads held above water only by their belief and trust in God.

Nancy Shoemaker, a psychiatric nurse, recounts a story of a patient diagnosed with bipolar disorder.

I worked with a forty-year-old woman who had a significant substance abuse history, which only complicated her bipolar disorder. She was preoccupied with her life mistakes and blamed herself without mercy. She felt particularly guilty about giving up her two children for adoption. I offered her nonjudgmental acceptance and praised her efforts to comply with treatment. I expressed faith in her ability to recover even with repeated slips. I also encouraged her to rely on her faith in God to learn to forgive herself. With the help of the psychiatric team, she attained sobriety, improved her mood, and made contact with her children.

Joyce Kistlinger, a community resource counselor, provided a very religious Christian woman with information about a prayer hotline: "The patient was very emotionally and spiritually needy. She had already shared with me the importance that her faith, and particularly prayer, played in her life. When I told her about the prayer hotline, she used it immediately and reported that this really had helped her."

In meeting the spiritual needs of psychiatric patients, it is imperative that we are continually aware and respectful of boundary issues, and never impose our spiritual beliefs on the patient.

Dr. Michael Parker ran a weekly group therapy session for nonpsychotic psychiatric patients in a day treatment program. He says, "The focus of the group was spirituality, and many of the participants shared negative experiences with organized religion. I was able to help them distinguish between religion and personal spirituality. This seemed to be helpful to them and their recovery."

Ada Scharf, a nurse, explains how her prayer and fasting has helped a friend with schizophrenia.

Recently I became concerned about a friend whom I had not seen for over a year. My friend is diagnosed with schizophrenia. Several years ago she had come to me asking for my help in distinguishing between hallucinations and demons. I didn't give her a good answer, nor did I refer her to someone who could help her. This bothered me. I began to pray and fast for her at regular times. Within a month of my prayer and fasting, my friend called me and asked to get together. We continue to have a friendship, and she shares her ups and downs with me. I encourage her to maintain her treatment, but I also encourage her weak faith by occasionally providing psychospiritual resources, Bible studies with strong mental health themes, and prayer guides.

REFLECTIONS

- Have you ever provided spiritual care to a patient with a psychiatric issue? What was the nature of that care?
- How would you go about respecting boundaries yet provide spiritual care?
- How can you communicate that research demonstrates that religion has a beneficial impact on psychiatric illness and respect the patient's boundaries?
- Reread Nancy Shoemaker's story. What are the spiritual needs of the patient Nancy describes? What were the spiritual interventions she offered?
- What circumstances would you consider before praying with a psychiatric patient?

DEMENTIA PATIENTS

Considering the fact that today over 4 million Americans are diagnosed with Alzheimer's disease (AD), and this number is expected to increase to 14 million by the year 2050,[9] healthcare providers must be prepared to provide whole-person care. This involves meeting the needs for physical and emotional care and managing challenging behaviors, as well as responding to the spiritual needs of this group.

Every aspect of life, including the spiritual, is altered when dementia afflicts a person. Confusion, limited judgment, decreased memory, physical losses, and decline in environmental mastery limit the dementia patient's ability to communicate. Working with a person who shows such limitations may lead to a sense of futility when considering how to meet spiritual needs. Some healthcare providers even take the position that the spiritual aspects of a confused person's life don't matter—the person won't understand anyway.

Healthcare professionals as well as lay caregivers must continue to believe that some things get through to the person with dementia even when response is limited. Long-term memory cradles religious beliefs and expressions of faith developed in early years. These memories can be tapped into long after short-term memory is gone and even into late-stage dementia.

Buckwalter reminds us:

Profound memory loss is associated with "loss of self"; however it never means loss of soul! . . . We must be aware of how memory loss leads to chaos in the soul. Our memories allow us to hold onto God's loving presence in our lives. We can trust God to be present to us in the here and now only because we remember the experience of God's presence and help in our past. The person with AD experiences a break in the very memories that provide continuity and connection to God that sustains most of us until our last breath. For a person with AD every day is new and everyone is a stranger—with no connection to the past, how can the person with AD experience that God will not abandon him? When one cannot remember who one is it is difficult to remember whose one is (God's) and to find comfort.[10]

Each of us who touch this patient's life—healthcare professionals and lay caregivers as well as the community of faith—have a responsibility to assist the person with AD to find his or her way home to God through the chaos and confusion of dementia. Alzheimer's patients may find God through their current experience of us, as we communicate God's love, kindness, and acceptance. God uses us to communicate his presence to these patients.

> A friend knows the song in my heart and sings it to me when my memory fails.
>
> —Author Unknown

This places an awesome responsibility on us. Each confused person remains a spiritually unique individual, and knowing what has been meaningful to the person and using this affirms that uniqueness. To carry out this responsibility and privilege, it is essential that we discover the patient's "meaning making" history. Conducting a spiritual history by asking family members about the patient's faith tradition, what religious rituals and practices were important, what activities brought joy to the person, and what place prayer, music, poetry, and faith symbols played in the person's life provides us with a foundation for meeting the dementia patient's spiritual needs by leading us to use religious music, symbols, and rituals to reach the patient.

Alternatively, the history may also lead us to use art, photography, and nature to make the connections. People with dementia continue to respond to visual aids such as candles, the Bible, a rosary, mezuzah, menorah, or a sculpture of praying hands; to sounds such as the recording of hymns, organs, the shofar horn, and words of Scripture and liturgy; and to aromas such as incense, fresh bread, and wine. These are all life-giving and provide bridges that assist the person with AD to reconnect with body and heart spiritual memories.

It is important to strengthen the pastoral connection that the patient has to his or her church, synagogue, mosque, or temple. A visit from a priest, minister, rabbi, or imam can provide powerful spiritual support. Reception of the sacraments remains an important spiritual event for patients with AD.

A nursing home assistant remembers taking care of an eighty-five-year-old woman who seemed to be totally nonresponsive. Every day the nursing assistant provided physical care to this woman's body; she talked to her patiently and with compassion; she gently brushed and braided her long hair; she massaged her back; and she made sure she was turned regularly and kept clean. None of these ministrations elicited a response. One day the nursing assistant was brushing the woman's hair, and as she worked, she began to sing the words to "Amazing Grace." Immediately this woman, who responded to nothing, began to move her lips as if she were singing along, and tears flowed down her cheeks. Had the nursing assistant touched this woman's soul?

REFLECTIONS

🕿 Have you taken care of patients suffering from dementia?

🕿 How do you think you could meet the spiritual needs of the patient with dementia?

🕿 What do you think about the use of prayer, Scripture, or religious music when you are unable to obtain validation from the patient that these interventions would be appreciated?

🕿 Reread the following quotation: "For a person with AD every day is new and everyone is a stranger—with no connection to the past, how can the person with AD experience that God will not abandon him? When one cannot remember who one is it is difficult to remember whose one is (God's) and to find comfort." What response does this elicit in you? How can you respond to this profound disconnection that occurs in AD?

CAREGIVERS

Another group of people who are deeply in need of spiritual support are those who provide care to incapacitated family members, including the caregivers of those with AD. For many who provide this care lovingly and generously, their decision to do so necessitates putting their own lives on hold. They push aside their own goals and desires to be available to meet the needs of someone else. Let there be no doubt that this is a difficult job. Many times the caregiving needs require 24/7 availability. Frequently, family members are called on to provide what is considered skilled nursing care in addition to meeting basic needs for nutrition and hydration, bathing, toileting, exercising, and comforting.

The job of caretaking can be physically and emotionally exhausting. It can also be spiritually depleting. Sometimes putting life in perspective is difficult. Healthcare providers must be aware of the physical, emotional, and spiritual toll that caregiving exacts and be prepared to address these areas of need. It might be helpful to suggest resources that provide spiritual sustenance. Such resources might include sacred scripture such as the Bible, Torah, or Koran.

If the caregiver finds it impossible to eke out a space for devotional reading, perhaps a beneficial alternative might be to read short passages to the patient/loved one. The Christian caregiver should be encouraged to read Matthew 25:34–36, bearing in mind that as she cares for the patient/loved one, it is as if she is caring for Jesus himself ("I was sick and you looked after me," verse 36), qualifying the caregiver to "take your inheritance, the kingdom prepared for you since the creation of the world" (verse 34, New International Version).

Familiar hymns, prayers, and poems can also sustain the caregiver's spirit as well as the spirit of the one needing care. Another important strategy for the caregiver is to stay connected to his or her faith community. This cuts down on the sense of isolation and emptiness that can result from total caregiving and might provide a support system that can relieve the burden.

Suggesting that the caregiver use journaling as a way of responding to spiritual issues is another potential intervention. Some approaches to journaling that may be helpful to caregivers include:

• Write about past memories of the loved one before caregiving days.

• List sources of gratitude, no matter how insignificant they may seem.

• Expand on memorable quotations from newspapers, magazines, or any other source.

• Inventory all the demanding roles of caregiving and offer self-congratulations for managing so many tasks.

• Write messages to God asking for help with particular situations.

It is important to include the date of all journal entries, plus other pertinent details such as the time of day, your location, and what you were doing. Rereading the journal entries fosters hope because frequently the writer recognizes how many challenges have been successfully handled.

Eileen Altenhofer, a parish nurse, shares her experience conducting a family support group.

One of my functions as a parish nurse is to co-facilitate a support group for family caregivers. The group is open to all in our community, and it is not disease specific. The attendees come from many different faith traditions, so it is not appropriate for me to discuss my own religious beliefs during the meeting. However, my co-leader and I still want to contribute to meeting the spiritual needs of family caregivers, who experience grief and deal with chronic and debilitating illness on a daily basis.

Drawing on my own spirituality, I close the meetings with a reflection based on the needs of the caregivers. I also make greeting cards with an uplifting quote or verse, which I think speaks to everyone. The members of the group take the card home. They may choose to display it on a bulletin board or a refrigerator, and it reminds them that they are in our hearts. Sometimes the members tell us that they give the card to the person that they are caring for, or send it to a friend in need. I am always touched by the response to the cards. Whatever quote or verse I have chosen, it seems to touch the soul of at least one of the members. One of the gentlemen told me how much his wife, whom he cares for, looks forward to receiving the cards.

Resources for spiritual sustenance can include sacred scripture such as the Bible, Torah, or Koran. If the caregiver finds it impossible to eke out a space for devotional reading, perhaps reading short passages to the patient/loved one might be uplifting. Familiar hymns, prayers, and poems can also sustain the caregiver's spirit as well as the spirit of the one needing care.

Another way that I think we meet the spiritual needs of the caregivers is to respectfully listen to their concerns and to offer information on resources that can help them. I feel that knowing there is help gives hope. If one has hope one can be more at peace. Hope replaces despair and gives a sense of direction. Providing information about available resources gives the feeling that the wider community cares and can be helpful.

REFLECTIONS

ᘘ What are your experiences working with caregivers?

ᘘ From your experience, what have you learned about their spiritual needs?

ᘘ How are you able to assist them to meet those needs?

PATIENTS WITH DEVASTATING INJURY

Patients who have experienced a devastating injury are also in need of spiritual support. The injury they have sustained may change their lives forever. It may affect their ability to function, their self-esteem, their body image, their sense of hope, their relationship to God, and their ability to pray. It would be easy for a healthcare provider to overlook the spiritual issues at the onset of the injury, where focus is on medical stabilization. Long-term care of the person with a devastating injury, however, must include a spiritual component. This is especially true when such an injury occurs to a young person.

Carole Kornelis, a parish nurse, prayed with an injured person:

One of the families in our faith community was involved in a car accident where the mother lost vision in her left eye due to a traumatic blow to the occipital area of the brain. Fear, anxiety, excruciating pain, and physical limitations wracked this poor woman's body. Since her two sons were also passengers in the vehicle, and remained absent from school for a few days, I made a home visit to determine needs. After a short visit and sensing the mother's despair and fear, I asked her if I could pray with her. She responded so positively and told me that she experienced a sense of peace that flooded her as a result of the prayer. She begged me to come back, and when I did, she took my hands and placed them on her head and asked me to pray.

REFLECTIONS

ᘘ What is your experience caring for a patient who experienced a traumatic injury?

🕸 Did spirituality play a role in the care of this patient?

🕸 What spiritual needs would you anticipate to be part of this clinical situation?

PATIENTS WHO NEED SURGERY

It is common for patients who are anticipating major surgery to feel anxious, fearful, and vulnerable. It is not only the patient who experiences this stress but the family as well.[11] They worry about the outcome of surgery. Patients and families are concerned about whether the patient will live or die. They worry about whether the surgery will correct whatever the medical problem is. They worry about whether the patient will be disabled or in pain as a result of the surgery. Retired ophthalmologist Dr. Gunnar E. Christiansen remembers, "Occasionally I would have a patient request that I pray with him during the preoperative visit. By doing so, I believe we were both given strength."

The most commonly used spiritual resource in preparation for surgery is prayer. In a study of 100 patients about to undergo cardiac surgery, 96 percent of the patients reported using prayer to deal with the stress of surgery, and 70 percent gave prayer the highest possible rating for helpfulness.[12] Prayer used before surgery helps relieve the stress, burden, and anxiety surrounding the anticipated procedure.

Surgical recovery may also benefit from prayer. In one study, frequent prayer to God was associated with greater compliance with the medical regimen.[13] In another study, prayer with chaplains was associated with 33 percent less use of pain medication in the postoperative period.[14]

Dr. Tom Grace, a plastic surgeon, sees the spiritual and religious needs of patients and families he meets every day.

I work in a Catholic hospital, where this aspect of care is addressed as part of care. Some of the interventions that I see and in which I participate include praying with patients before surgery. Regardless of the reason for surgery, whether for a serious or a minor condition, the prospect of surgery makes patients anxious. They fear bad outcomes; they fear the anesthesia; they feel the anticipated pain after surgery. At the bottom of this is a fear of death. Many patients and families ask for prayer and receive it with no hesitation—not only from me, but also from the nuns and priests who circulate through the hospital throughout the day and evening and come into the preoperative and the recovery area. They add to what I can provide by offering prayer, comfort, and their presence.

Sandra Brown, an advanced practice nurse, remembers taking care of a Jewish postoperative patient who was frightened and alone and hurting about family issues. "I drew on my knowledge of Jewish beliefs that speak of God and the Old Testament picture of his being with her. I referred to the Patriarchs and their faith and encouraged her that God was in complete control and that she could trust the God of her ancestors. She was deeply appreciative."

REFLECTIONS

&* Have you ever had surgery? What were your concerns? How did you use your spiritual resources to deal with your concerns?

&* What is your experience in providing spiritual assistance to patients preparing for surgery?

&* Reread Dr. Grace's statement about the importance of prayer before surgery. What are your reactions to what he says? What is your role in facilitating prayer before surgery?

CHILDREN

The last group of patients to be considered is sick children. Not only does the child have needs for spiritual support, but the parents do as well. Healthcare providers must be attuned to these spiritual needs and be willing to meet them through presence, actions, and words.

Pediatric nurse Carole Richards is able to meet spiritual needs through kindness and gentleness:

I once received a note from a mother of a child for whom I had provided care. She wrote, "You sat beside our daughter, holding her hand, massaging her hand and arm, and singing to her. You washed her hair and brought her out of her room where she could see other people. Because we had seen the consistent gentle and loving care you gave while we were there, we were able to leave her in your hands with real peace of mind whenever we had to leave the hospital. Respite also came in the form of the calming effect you had on everyone in our family. If you were ever rattled, we certainly didn't know it! Your trust in God to help you handle the difficult situations facing you encouraged us to also trust him." This kind of sums up the ways that I try to provide spiritual care to all the children and parents I encounter.

REFLECTIONS

🕮 Have you ever taken care of a sick child? If so, what spiritual needs did you assess? How did you respond to these needs?

🕮 Do you have children? If so, have you ever experienced the serious illness of one of your children? What were your child's spiritual needs? What were yours? Did any healthcare provider respond to those needs? How would you have wanted a healthcare provider to respond?

We have examined spiritual care across many different clinical situations. Now let's turn our attention to providing spiritual care for ourselves. How do we nurture our own spirits so that we have resources to draw upon when we are confronted with the needs of our patients? Chapter 9 explores this topic.

[9]

Nurturing the Self
Nurturing the Spirit

> *Like our patients, we are also exhorted to rejoice in our sufferings,*
> *in the privilege of sharing the burden. We are to rejoice not only in*
> *giving but in receiving the healing love of the community. That*
> *love can empower in us, too, the endurance that can produce a*
> *character full of hope in the love that does not allow suffering to*
> *divide us. This is where we find our healing: where our work is,*
> *where our love acts.*
> —Dr. Margaret E. Mohrmann, *Medicine as Ministry*

We have heard the stories of doctors, nurses, therapists, counselors, social workers, healthcare administrators, health educators, and chaplains. Many shared with us that spirituality is not only essential to their work but that it drives what they do. They believe that their work is much more than a job; it is a ministry of compassion. How do these caregivers maintain their own spiritual health? Can they continue to give without replenishing their personal spiritual reserves? What activities are spiritually nurturing?

This chapter examines the necessity for all of us to consciously seek out and plan activities that feed our souls—that restock what we give and keep us connected to and grounded in our God.

RECIPROCITY OF CAREGIVING

According to Mohrmann,[1] those who minister to the sick and suffering are required to give of themselves, their knowledge, time, faith, passion, and strength—without stopping. The giving needs to be exuberant and extravagant with no stinginess or holding back, all in the service of love. This does not mean that as healthcare providers we are so tied to work that we never leave the workplace. There are others who need our time and our love—families, friends, neighbors, and faith communities all have valid claims on our extravagant love. We are not God; we are finite human beings who live within the boundaries of time and bodies that require rest. Nor are we to give in to a belief that if we extravagantly love those who suffer, we will have nothing left for others whom we love. It is one of life's greatest paradoxes: the more love we give to others without expectation of return, the more we have to give.

There are days, however, when we may feel drained with nothing more to share. We may want to pull away and protect ourselves from the never-ending stream of suffering people who walk through our lives looking for care and compassion. We may feel empty and unable to draw one more drop of compassion from our lamp of love. At these times, however, it is important to distinguish between fatigue and emptiness. It is easy to confuse being spiritually empty with being too tired to give. We need to be good stewards of finite energy and time—recognizing and honoring our limitations. Operating with an energy deficit is not the same as having a love deficit.[2]

If indeed we are drained of love, then we must also consider that perhaps we have stopped receiving from God. Perhaps we have allowed every moment of our day to be filled with commitments to others, leaving us with no quiet time or no time for just being in God's presence and receiving his overflowing love. Perhaps we have built blockades that keep us from receiving the love that is available to us from family and friends, and from our own self-care. Physician Christina Puchalski recognizes that keeping a commitment to be present to patients, families, and colleagues draws on spiritual resources that require periodic restoration. She tries to schedule occasional home workdays where she can retreat from the hectic schedule and constant demands of working in a university-hospital setting. She also seeks renewal time in spiritual retreats where the focus is on quieting the soul and receiving God's refreshment.

Just as important as our discernment regarding fatigue and emptiness is awareness that we can be refilled by the very people to whom we are giving. The very people we are called to love, those people we are called to heal, are givers as well as receivers. As wounded healers, we need to recognize that we are in a reciprocal relationship with those we serve. It is important to acknowledge that those same sufferers, even when they are most in need of receiving from us, can still give. To deny this is to deny them the opportunity to participate in full personhood and to enter into relation with us.

In what ways do the sufferers give back to us and show us mercy? First, they allow us to love and to serve. They provide us with opportunities to live out our God-given purpose and responsibility and to feel that our lives have deep meaning. They allow us to enter into their worlds—to hear their stories—to participate in and even to affect their lives' journeys.

Patients provide us with opportunities to live out our God-given purpose and to feel that our lives have deep meaning. They allow us to enter into their worlds—to hear their stories—to participate in and even to affect their lives' journeys. Our patients teach us how to perfect our roles as healers.

Second, our patients are teachers. They teach us how to perfect our roles as healers. They teach us how to take professional knowledge and, in the process of applying this knowledge, make it come alive in the context of human life and suffering. They teach us far more than the manifestations of various diagnoses; they teach us the nature of their illnesses and what it means to suffer.

Third, our patients provide structure to our own stories. They contribute many of the rich details that are woven together to form the tapestry of our lives.

Those who are called to be healers, to be healthcare providers and ministers, are called not only to give but also to receive from God and from the ones whom they serve. This, as Mohrmann puts it, is the "music of God's essential dance of love—freely receive, freely give."[3]

REFLECTIONS

- As you think about your practice, have there been times when you confused being tired for being empty?
- How do you balance the demands on your time and love?
- As you reflect on your practice, in what ways do the very patients you serve also sustain you?
- How have patients taught you how to be better in your role as a healing practitioner?
- How have patients provided you some of the threads of your life's tapestry?
- What weavings stand out on that tapestry?
- How have you participated in God's dance of love?

EXPRESSIONS OF SPIRIT

Spirit is a difficult word to define. It is elusive, subjective, and hard to grasp. Definitions seem too ethereal and lacking in objectivity. Yet when we talk about spirit, most people understand what is meant. Spirit is like the wind that rustles through the leaves and blows a gentle breeze across our faces. Sometimes it is gentle; at other times it can be incredibly forceful. We see the results of spirit—we feel its presence and influence, but we cannot grasp it in our hands, nor can we contain it. We are painfully aware of the absence of spirit and many times describe those who are feeling sad as being in "low spirits." Conversely, we might describe an exuberant individual as being "high spirited."

As healthcare professionals, we might intervene if we assessed that someone was so low spirited as to be considered clinically depressed. We would be correct to intervene, because sometimes a person's spirits become so desperately low that they lack the spirit to desire life. Thoughts of suicide are as much a spiritual problem as they are a psychiatric symptom. When a person seriously considers and plans suicide, what that person is saying is this: "No one cares whether I live or die—no one, not even God." When a person is disheartened enough to believe their life is worthless to everyone, including God, then suicide becomes a viable alternative. Such low spirits are life threatening and require outside intervention to bolster the individual until their own spirit level is increased and depression is decreased.[4]

Dr. Ruth Stoll, nurse-author, proposes a number of definitions of spirit:[5]

• The image of God within every person, making one a thinking, feeling, moral, creative being able to relate meaningfully to God (as defined by that person), self, and others
• A human drive to bond with the transcendent
• An animating, life-giving dimension that transcends all other dimensions of the person
• The literal breath of life
• The real person, the part of us nobody can see, the part that doesn't die . . . the inside you . . .
• Provides people the capacity to be conscious of God

REFLECTIONS

❧ How do you define "spirit"?

❧ How do you know when a patient is in "low spirits"? Is there a difference between clinical depression and spiritual distress? If so, how would you differentiate the two?

❧ What are the signs that you are feeling low spirited? How do you behave? What do you do to raise your spirits?

WHAT DEPLETES OUR SPIRITS?

Sometimes we allow busyness and commitments to totally consume us to the point that there is no time for spiritual refueling. We risk experiencing spiritual burnout. We feel exhausted and empty, and we begin to ask questions such as, Is there a compelling *why* for what I do and who I am? Do I make a difference? Why am I suffering when I give so much? Is there a purpose to this suffering? What more does God want from me? These questions symbolize a crisis of meaning. We are like a tire without a wheel—we lack a center that gives us direction. We feel lost, and spiritual renewal is important in helping us to find our way back to our center.

Periodically, it is a good idea to take stock regarding how we spend our time. It is important to inventory those activities that make us feel spiritually alive as well as those activities that diminish our spirits. What are the sources of spirit depletion?

> Is there a compelling *why* for what I do and who I am? Do I make a difference? Why am I suffering when I give so much? Is there a purpose to this suffering? What more does God want from me? These questions symbolize a crisis of meaning.

Not Knowing We Are God's Beloved

Catholic theologian Henri Nouwen was asked by a Jewish friend and journalist, Fred Bratman, to write a book for secular men and women who wonder what life is all about but lack religious convictions and beliefs to guide them.[6] Bratman challenged Nouwen to speak to those who were outside traditional religious systems and who lacked the language to appreciate religious metaphors and teachings. Bratman told Nouwen, "Speak to us about the deepest yearnings of our hearts, about our many wishes, about hope; not about the many strategies for survival, but about trust; not about new methods of satisfying our emotional needs, but about love. Speak to us about a vision larger than our changing perspectives and about a voice deeper than the clamorings of our mass media. Yes, speak to us about something or someone greater than ourselves. Speak to us about . . . God."[7]

Nouwen accepted Bratman's challenge and wrote the book *Life of the Beloved: Spiritual Living in a Secular World*. In this book Nouwen asserts that the major obstacle to living spiritually is that we cannot conceive that anyone, certainly not God, considers us beloved. Our minds are filled with our own negative voices that tell us all that is wrong with us. We ask ourselves, "How can we be anyone's beloved until we can straighten ourselves out and engage in serious self-improvement?"

We fall into a trap of self-rejection that, according to Nouwen, is the greatest enemy of the spiritual life because it contradicts the sacred voice. Self-rejection pushes us to spend too much time listening to a voice that shouts at us to prove we are worth something, that demands that we engage in only relevant and important activities, that convinces us that by ourselves we are unworthy of love, and that love is not freely given, only earned. We spend a great deal of our lives trying to be better and to do more. We tell ourselves, "If only I could . . . I would be loved."

Meanwhile, the soft, gentle voice that speaks to us in the silence of our hearts and considers us beloved remains unheard. So we look to our jobs, our patients, our families and friends, our accomplishments, and other outward signs for proof that we are worthy and lovable. We ignore the voice of God who calls to us:

I have called you by name, from the very beginning. You are mine and I am yours. You are my Beloved, on you my favor rests. I have molded you in the depths of the earth and knitted you together in your mother's womb. I have carved you in the palms of my hands and hidden you in the shadow of my embrace. I look at you with infinite tenderness and care for you with a care more intimate than that of a mother for her child. I have counted every hair on your head and guided you at every step. Wherever you go, I go with you, and wherever you rest, I keep watch. I will give you food that will satisfy all your hunger and drink that will quench all your thirst. I will not hide my face from you. You know me as your own and I know you as my own. You belong to me. I am your father, your mother, your brother, your child . . . wherever you are I will be. Nothing will ever separate us.[8]

If we really believe we are God's beloved, we begin to look to God for comfort, for restoration, and for guidance—knowing full well that God's love is completely unconditional. He doesn't love us more today because of some great personal accomplishment; he won't love us less tomorrow because we are the source of pain or disappointment for someone else. The whole notion of being loved for who we are—for just *being*—is almost more than our minds can handle. Perhaps it is only for our hearts and spirits to embrace. But embracing this truth frees us to give generously, to love extravagantly, to feel joy beyond comprehension. Why? Because God loves us. When we forget this core truth we stumble, we try to fix things ourselves, we accept responsibility for everything, and we hurt.

Many of those that we interviewed commented on the importance of staying in God's presence. Retired physician Gunnar Christiansen described this most eloquently.

We ignore the voice of God who calls to us, "I have called you by name, from the very beginning. You are mine and I am yours." Instead, we listen to the inner voice that shouts at us to prove we are worth something, that demands that we engage in only relevant and important activities, that convinces us that by ourselves we are unworthy of love—that love is not freely given, only earned.

I believe my spirituality is God working in me as well as being part of me. Through meditation and prayer, my sense of God's presence is increased. Likewise, my awareness of my ability and my opportunity to have God assist me in my attempts to use my gifts in the service of others is increased. Maintaining my spiritual health or direction has not been consistent or easy. In those times that I focus too much on myself and not enough on others, my sense of peace in the presence of God is significantly reduced. Nevertheless, my sense of God's forgiving love when I return to him with my pleas for forgiveness and strength enables me to continue to attempt to follow a pathway that appears to be his will.

Being Diminished

Another source of spiritual distress is the experience of being made to feel small. This is closely linked to not knowing we are beloved by God. Almost everyone we interviewed, across all healthcare professions, commented on the critical importance for people to feel affirmed in what they do. The consensus was that lack of affirmation was closely related to a high turnover rate.

It is important for healthcare providers to know that they make a difference, that they are appreciated, and that they are cared about. Martha Loveland, healthcare administrator, believes that the most critical element of a spiritual work environment is that people are valued as God's creations. Harriet Coeling, nursing faculty member at Kent State University, asserts that the main reasons nurses leave a job situation or leave nursing completely is a lack of respect from those to whom they report, a lack of appreciation for what they do, and unreasonable working conditions.

Meaningless Work

So much of what we do in healthcare is embedded with deep meaning. However, in addition to the meaningful and rewarding aspects of patient care, there is a mountain of required paperwork, government regulations such as HIPAA compliance, regulatory issues, and insurance requirements—so much that it makes healthcare providers want to throw up their hands in despair and shout, Enough! Many painfully concede that the amount of paperwork required drastically reduces the amount of time that is available to care for people. Sometimes it seems as if the chart is more important than the patient.

The most critical element of a spiritual work environment is that people are valued as God's creations.

Life Out of Balance

Maintaining a healthy balance in life is no easy feat—especially for people who are in caregiving roles. Because they have the skills to relieve pain and suffering and to make others feel better, they are constantly in demand. They may come to feel that everyone wants something from them. And it is not only patients and families, it is the rest of life that impinges on their time and their resources. How does anyone balance the demands of work, loving relationships, time for fun, quiet time with God, time for rest, and time for community activities? There is no easy answer. Everyone must find their own balance. What works comfortably for one person would feel like overload to someone else.

We must learn to listen to our bodies, our hearts, and our spirits. When we are out of balance—if we listen carefully enough, we will get the message—we will experience physical dysfunction, emotional problems, and/or a sense of distance from God. It is important that we heed those signals and take action to correct the imbalance. All of us can manage periods of imbalance, for instance when the end is in sight for completion of a major project. When the pattern of our lives is always out of balance, however, we will pay a steep price—physically, emotionally, and spiritually.

When we asked Chaplain Robb Small what he does to maintain his spiritual health, he replied, "Play often. A well-balanced life is important. I have learned to find ways of leaving my work and going away for mental- and spiritual-health time. I attend to my family and church, I pursue relationships with people outside my family that offer me meaning and purpose, and I look for things in life that help me maintain hope."

Always Being the Caretaker

It is important for us to remember that just as we give to patients and in return we receive from them, it is equally important that we are able to receive care and compassion from others. We may become accustomed to ignoring our own pain and suffering because there always seems to be someone who has greater needs than we do. But we don't always have to be the givers. Sometimes it is important and necessary for the well-being of our bodies and souls to be receivers. All of us need to be cared for; all of us need to know that someone is concerned about us. All of us need to know that God will care for us—but we have to let him.

SPIRITUAL INVENTORY

How do I feel about myself as a healthcare provider?

What are the things that cause me the most stress?

As I look back on my life to date, what do I consider my greatest accomplishment?

What makes me the happiest?

How do I replenish my spirit?

When was the last time I did something just for myself? Something that made my spirits soar? That delighted my soul?

If I knew that I had only a brief time to live, what changes would I want to make in my life?

REFLECTIONS

⌘ In what ways does your life reflect that you are God's beloved?

⌘ What effect does it have on your spirit when you are diminished and made to feel small and inadequate? Does this experience get in the way of providing spiritual care to others?

⌘ Is your life in balance? If not, what could you do to establish a healthy rhythm among the many demands of your life?

⌘ Are you usually/always the caretaker? What is your reaction to being the recipient of care? If you resist care from others, can you be open to receiving care from God?

FEEDING THE SPIRIT

Individuals develop different ways of nurturing their spirits. Some of these expressions derive from faith traditions, such as attendance at and participation in worship services; receiving communion; meditating; fasting; saying the rosary; wearing a prayer shawl; singing; reading the Torah, the Bible, or the Koran; and reaching out to others. Many of our participants mentioned the importance of attending Sunday worship services, going to Mass, attending synagogue services, going to the mosque for Friday afternoon prayer, and participating in regular scripture-study groups.

Prayer is probably the most universal of spiritual expressions. In a 2001 national survey conducted by the Gallup Organization of 729 adults, 65 percent of Americans agreed (20 percent) or strongly agreed (45 percent) that they spend time in worship or prayer every day.[9] According to this report, "Some individuals begin their day with half an hour of devotional reading followed by silent prayer; others end their day with meditation and reading from a prayer book; still others listen to inspirational tapes or CDs in their car and use their morning or evening commute as a time of reflection. Some individuals do this alone, preferring solitude in their quest for spiritual growth. Others share their daily prayer time with another person or group of people."

In this same poll, participants were asked if they use prayer instead of getting medical treatment, use prayer in addition to getting medical treatment, or never use prayer. Sixty-seven percent reported using prayer in a medical context, while 31 percent said they never used prayer in such a context. Furthermore, 25 percent of Americans reported having personally asked someone else to pray for them to help cure a medical condition in the past twelve months.

With regard to the prayer lives of health professionals in general, we know very little from systematic research. There are a few studies, however, that shed some light on this area. For instance, in one study of 39 nurses and 130 physicians at Duke Hospital, participants were asked to what extent their religious beliefs helped with coping (where religious coping primarily involved praying).[10] Among nurses, 67 percent indicated "a large extent or more"; among physicians, 41.7 percent indicated this response. The biggest difference was in the extent to which these health professionals depended on their religious beliefs as "the most important factor that keeps you going": 25.6 percent of nurses indicated this was true, whereas only 8.7 percent of physicians did so.

Another study of 1,221 physicians, nurses, physical therapists, and occupational therapists who specialize in physical medicine and rehabilitation also found that nurses and occupational therapists were more likely to pray than physicians and physical therapists.[11]

In a study of nurses, Marsh and colleagues found that 67 percent of the nurses strongly agreed that prayer was an important part of their lives, and 56 percent noted that prayer was important to them in making decisions.[12] Still another study of 142 nurses (78 percent), physicians (11 percent), nurse practitioners (3 percent), and other healthcare professionals (7 percent), nearly two thirds (65.5 percent) indicated that they used prayer or spiritual practices for the promotion of their own health and well-being.[13]

Everyone who participated in this book commented on the central role of prayer in their spiritual lives. Many noted the importance of both speaking to God and allowing God to speak to them during prayer time. It is not enough to pour out our hearts to God. Solid relationships require two-way communication. It is essential that we allow God to speak to our hearts and souls and to flood us with his grace and wisdom. Such a conversation is essential if we are doing God's work. It only makes sense that we stay in touch with the boss! Martha Loveland, healthcare administrator, says, "I set aside a small physical place in my home for daily prayer and meditation. I play special music during this time. It is important that I make prayer a focal point of every day."

Creative expressions through music, the arts, and storytelling may allow connection with God's refreshing and restorative love. Several of our participants mentioned the importance of music. Charmin Koenig, a former X-ray technician and nurse, listens to Christian music throughout the day and volunteers her services at a local Christian radio station. "Music is so important to me," she says. "It keeps me calm and focused on the Lord all day. I can't be without music." Family practice physician Bernita Taylor also comments on the importance of music to her soul: "I sing with the Swarthmore College Alumni Gospel Choir. I graduated in 1980 and have known many of the members since my student days. They are family to me."

Everyday activities may also provide a transcendent opportunity to link with God as we think about why we are engaging in this mundane task. Preparing school lunches for children, for example, can be more than just a chore. As the mother reflects on the gift of her children, packing a lunch becomes an act of love and thanksgiving.

Occupational therapist Jay Brashear describes the transformation of another ordinary activity: "When I am assisting a patient with bathing, I imagine that I am providing this service to the Lord himself. For me, there is power in this thinking. It changes my attitude and my way of relating. My approach then is no longer about completing the bath. It is all about how this bath is conveying love."

Relationships are also a source of spiritual renewal, and many of the participants commented on the support that they gain from family, friends, their faith community, and those to whom they provide care.

Charmin Koenig is active in her church's women's ministry and says her spirit is fed by serving.

Eileen Altenhofer, a parish nurse, talks about the importance of spending time with her partner in parish nurse ministry.

I walk with a special friend, Joan Wieringa, and we affirm one another in our conversations. I share my concerns with close family and friends. I pursue my passions—artwork with use of the computer and time with my grandchildren. My grandson meets my spiritual needs on a most deep level. He is only seven, but he has the sweet, innocent faith of a child. Once I asked him how many people were at a party he attended. He listed the people and then said, "and God." I think I looked a little startled at his response, because he fixed his gaze on me and said, "Now, Grandma, you know God is always with us."

Charity Johansson observes that an important aspect of taking care of her spiritual health is to talk and listen to wise people: "It is the most consistent and most powerful part of how I feed my spirit. Every day I find time to spend with someone who is willing to converse in depth and to join me in the search for meaning."

Other people find God in the beauty of his creation. Kelly Preston loves to run. During her runs she enjoys the outdoors, feels invigorated, clears her mind, and listens to God.

Shirley Herron describes her reaction to seeing an iceberg off of the coast of St. Johns, Newfoundland.

My friend and I stood on the shore of the Atlantic Ocean mesmerized by two magnificent icebergs just off the coast. These pristine white shapes dwarfed the boats that circled around them. The waves lapped against the edges, eroding the iceberg as it touched the ocean's surface, bringing out a beautiful turquoise color that reflected the sun.

As we stood contemplating the beauty of these icebergs, it occurred to me how similar they were to the uniqueness and wonder of each person that we encounter in Spiritual Direction. Underneath the surface of the water is a supporting structure approximately ten times the size of the visible berg. I thought of this visible part of the iceberg as representing the persona of each of us, that part that we pres-

ent to the world, even to those who know us well. Underneath is the real self with all of its joys and dreams, wounds and uncertainties. As the waves of the ocean lap against the surface of the iceberg, it melts away the upper structure, and a part of the iceberg "calves" away, falling forever into the ocean and disappearing. As this occurs, I believe part of the "real iceberg" lifts a little, exposing itself to the visible eye.

Then I realized that the iceberg was suspended, immersed, supported by the vast ocean in which it floated. We are similarly immersed in the incomprehensible love of God. Our true self is supported and sustained in that love. All of our wounded, aching places are always being lapped by God's love. God's desire is to "calve" away the false persona and reveal the beauty of the true self as he has created us, and to heal the wounded places.

I saw the iceberg in sunshine and in deep fog. The circumstances made no difference; the iceberg was always supported by the sea. Sometimes the waves were gentle and sometimes not. Still the iceberg was embraced by the sea. Whatever the circumstance of our lives, we are still enfolded in God's love. It is our natural environment, as the sea is the natural environment for the iceberg.

REFLECTIONS

⳾ What do you do to replenish your spirit?

⳾ As you reflect on your years in healthcare, have you ever experienced a crisis of meaning? What were the circumstances of your life at that time? How did you move to a place of wholeness again?

⳾ Are there rituals or practices from your faith tradition that are particularly meaningful to you?

⳾ Are there other nonreligious activities that feed your spirit?

We know that caregiving can be both rewarding and life-giving as well as frustrating and life-draining. The difference depends on whether we seek to nurture our own spirits. There is no way around it—we cannot continue giving without receiving. Spiritual restoration is possible through prayer, worship, devotional reading, relationships, nature, music, and the arts. (See Appendix C for additional resources to support spiri-tuality.)

Ultimately, though, the in-filling of our spirits must come from God, and that requires us to pull away from the demands of work, family life, and other commitments to spend time in God's presence. Throughout all the world's great religions, we see examples of pulling back from ser-vice to spend time with God. In Scripture we see the example of Moses drawing back from the Israelites to speak to God; we see Jesus separat-ing himself from his apostles to spend time with his Father in prayer; Mohammed often went off by himself to pray to Allah; Buddha was said to spend much time in meditation. We may argue that we don't have the time, that it is impossible for us to get away. If this is the case, then it is imperative to find the time. Our very spirits depend upon it.

Move on with us to the last chapter to examine where we go from here. How do we reclaim the vision of healthcare as a ministry? What, if anything, can we do as individuals to change the system? What can we do as groups of committed individuals of faith to change the system?

[10]

A David-and-Goliath Match

Taking On the System

*Never doubt that a small group of thoughtful, committed
citizens can change the world. Indeed it is the only thing that
ever has.*

—Margaret Mead

Throughout this book, we listened as healthcare providers shared
their stories of ministry to patients and families—always focusing on the
"caring" aspect of caregiving. We heard healthcare providers from many
different faith traditions describe the call they received from God to
enter their chosen professions. We listened as they described the ways
they live out that call every day. We listened as they described what they
do as more than a job but as collaborative work with and for God. We
heard their frustration as they described a healthcare system that is broken—that seems to subordinate human needs to economic concerns.
We listened as they described the devastating effects of working in this
broken healthcare system: healthcare providers as well as patients and
families feeling uncared for and diminished, employees experiencing job

dissatisfaction and leaving their positions, and priority being given to paperwork and profit rather than to patients.

WHAT CAN BE DONE?

This brings us to the final issue: Is there anything that can be done to make the system a spiritually healthy environment? Most people's first response is probably a resounding "No!" The system is too big, and the problems run too deep. We encourage each of you, however, to rethink that no. It is probably true that none of us can take on the whole system. It is too much—it is too overwhelming. But individuals can make a difference, and groups of like-minded individuals can change the system.

Let's start with the story of a system change that occurred because of one person's efforts.

In 1990, the homecare regulations specified that only psychiatrists were able to refer patients for psychiatric homecare services. This was a major problem, because many of the elderly receive treatment for depression and anxiety from internists as well as family and general practitioners. Many elderly believe being diagnosed with any psychiatric problem, such as depression, is a sign of character weakness and feel that they should be able to "pull themselves up by their bootstraps." Unfortunately, their bootstraps are frequently defective. A common reaction among the elderly is that seeing a psychiatrist means they are crazy.

Medicare's position that only psychiatrists should refer limited access to psychiatric homecare services. Troubled by having to turn away patients who needed psychiatric homecare services because there was no referring psychiatrist, a concerned individual, a psychiatric home health provider, wrote a letter requesting a personal appointment with Thomas Hoyer, who until 2003 held a leadership role in the Medicare administration. The appointment was granted, and the concerned individual presented a number of clinical situations where psychiatric homecare would have been the appropriate modality, but because the referring physician was not a psychiatrist, the service was denied. Mr. Hoyer acknowledged the validity of these arguments and said that if other home health providers would write or call him to express a similar sentiment, then change would come about.

So for the next year, the concerned individual, who spoke nationally, gave out Mr. Hoyer's telephone and fax numbers to thousands of home health providers and encouraged them to call him or to fax him a letter regarding this issue. At the end of the year, Mr. Hoyer's assistant called the individual to say, "Enough, we get the message! The regulation will be changed with the next revision of the HM-11" (Medicare's Home Care Regulations). In May 1996, the revision was released; it allows nonpsychiatrists to make referrals for psychiatric homecare. One person *can* make a difference!

IDENTIFY YOUR PASSION—INVENTORY YOUR GIFTS

But what can we do? The first step is to identify what we feel passionate enough about that we are willing to make a commitment to change—in ourselves, in our place of employment, in the system. We need to inventory our gifts. Some of us are excellent clinicians. Others are good writers. Others are excellent organizers of ideas, time, resources, and people. Still others are great at delegating. Others may be leaders, able to motivate and unite others to work toward change. Some are effective speakers who can inspire others through powerful oratory. Others may be researchers, striving to add to the body of knowledge that exists about the value of spiritual care. Others are innovators, trying to find new ways to improve patient care. Some are teachers, able to convey knowledge in a stimulating and exciting manner.

Each of us needs to identify his or her gifts and begin to use those gifts in a deliberate and thoughtful manner that benefits more than the patient and family seeking care, casting a wider net of influence.

THE POWER OF WORDS

Let's look at ways to cast our net of influence to reap broad change. We know that it is inappropriate to preach or proselytize to patients, families, or co-workers. We should never try to coerce others into believing as we do. Ideally, our *actions* should convey that we are spiritual individuals and that we are open to accepting and supporting the spirituality of others. Words, however, are powerful; words have the potential to encourage, influence, change, and even revolutionize! People tend to mull over the words of a conversation again and again, extracting different levels of meaning each time. Words carefully and deliberately spoken may hold sway over the listener years after the conversation has occurred.

For instance, taking a spiritual history/assessment sends an unmistakable message—not only to the patient and family, but also to fellow healthcare providers—that we believe this is an important part of the care, and we are willing to talk about it. Similarly, if the patient asks, it is appropriate to make "I" statements about our own beliefs and practices that let others know that we believe in God, we are people of faith, we pray and believe in the power of prayer, and we think spiritual issues are very important. Perhaps a patient or co-worker is confronted with a difficult, even life-threatening, situation and asks for advice and specifically wants to know what you would do. It is appropriate to say, "I think I would pray about it." A simple statement—a profession of faith, if you will—but a powerful statement. Such a statement does not tell the person what they should or ought to do, but very simply states what you would do.

When we combine caring actions with occasional, well-placed words of faith, we have delivered an incredibly effective intervention, and we are acting to spread the word.

This is not to say, however, that only people of faith are capable of utilizing a patient's spiritual resources to help that person. About ten years ago, Rebecca Propst led a research study comparing the effects of religious cognitive-behavioral therapy (CBT) and secular CBT on the treatment of depression in religious patients.[1] Each therapy was delivered by both secular and religious therapists. She and her colleagues found that those who received religious CBT improved more quickly than those who received secular CBT. Most surprising, however, was that the patients receiving religious CBT who got better the fastest were those who received CBT from *nonreligious secular* therapists.

THE POWER OF THE PEN

Writing is another way to spread the message about spiritual care. Many places of employment publish an employee newsletter that most likely includes a combination of informational articles, a forum to update employees about changes, and a place to acknowledge the achievements of employees. An article written about personal experiences obtaining spiritual assessments, detailing the difference this information makes to the plan of care, and the impact that seeking this information has on relationships with patients and families could influence professional colleagues. Or perhaps a series of articles could be written on the importance of spiritual care to patient outcomes.

Moving beyond the place of employment to the larger community might lead one to investigate submitting an article to a local newspaper. Frequently newspapers solicit articles on health-related and human interest topics. An article or a series of articles on spiritual care certainly fits both these categories. Spreading the word about spirituality beyond one's local community might involve submitting an article to a professional journal that has the potential to influence thousands of other healthcare professionals.

THE POWER OF KNOWLEDGE

Conducting research is a phenomenal strategy to make a difference in the area of spiritual care. Research on religion/spirituality and healthcare gives credence to the importance of spiritual care. Large research projects are usually funded by external sources that also convey credibility to the issues being investigated.

Science is built on the systematic accumulation of evidence—one research study building on another until a body of knowledge is established that irrefutably proves a certain point. In turn, health policy and reimbursement decisions are influenced by research findings. Research examining the impact of religion/spirituality on health outcomes is increasing exponentially and building that body of knowledge. The results of such studies are usually published in refereed journals as well as lay publications, so that the findings are disseminated to a wide audience. The findings may also be shared at conferences attended by healthcare professionals and the lay public. Research is clearly a way to cast the net of influence.

Where does this leave most of us who are not researchers? We may lack the skill, time, or inclination to be a researcher. We may feel overwhelmed by the work that goes into planning and implementing an effective research protocol. Those of us who are not researchers may be able to wield influence in our places of employment to seek participation in a research study on spirituality or to implement research findings in practice and training. This provides an avenue to contribute to knowledge without being totally responsible for the processes involved.

THE POWER OF ONE TO MULTIPLY

Let's return to the idea of taking a spiritual history/assessment and examine how individual efforts can be used to influence others to improve patient care. Those of us who are stepping out and performing spiritual histories/assessments and providing spiritual care need to talk about it. We need to be examples to other health professionals who are feeling unsure or uneasy about incorporating spiritual care into their practice.

Those of us who have leadership skills need to lead, because people listen to and emulate what a good leader suggests. We need to assume leadership in effecting practice standards. For instance, approaching the practice committee of our hospital or clinic would be an appropriate place to begin. A presentation encompassing the following three points would make a pretty powerful argument for the need to mandate spiritual care: (1) personal experiences of actually obtaining spiritual histories/assessments; (2) information on the JCAHO standard mandating spiritual assessments on patients in a general hospital, psychiatric patients, patients in long-term care, and patients receiving homecare; and (3) the results of a few well-selected research studies demonstrating the clinical and cost effectiveness of addressing spiritual needs.

Perhaps these efforts could lead to the development of a leadership

team consisting of influential health professionals and hospital administrators who recognize the importance of changing the system to include
spiritual care. This team could then design an educational program that
circumvents the resistance and barriers now present in the healthcare
system that are preventing spiritual integration. This educational intervention would encompass all health professionals at every level and
would provide instruction about the value and importance of meeting
patients' spiritual needs. Without a doubt, implementation of such an
educational effort would result in patient satisfaction, provider satisfaction, positive health outcomes, and perhaps even a decrease in the costs
associated with care.

EXPANDING THE DREAM

Let's look at two scenarios, one located in Pleasantville in which an
educational intervention took place, and one located in Drearytown in
which it did not.

In the hospital where the educational intervention took place, a
physician takes a spiritual history and uncovers a patient's spiritual
needs. Although this adds 1.2 minutes to the visit, the doctor-patient
relationship is enhanced, and trust develops. The patient is satisfied with
the doctor and the care delivered, and the doctor feels satisfied because
he or she seems to have truly helped this patient.

Since nurses are also required to address spiritual issues, the nurse
reads the spiritual history documented in the record by the physician
and asks the patient spiritual questions that might have a bearing on
nursing care. Nurses and/or social workers then assist to mobilize spiritual resources (including a visit with the chaplain, the patient's clergy or
parish nurse, and/or members of the patient's faith community) to help
the patient cope with illness during hospitalization and after discharge.
The healthcare team holds a care conference to discuss the spiritual
needs of the patient and a plan for meeting these needs. Individual
providers on the team are assigned roles as appropriate in this care.

As a result, patients cope better due to the spiritual support provided during and after hospitalization, recover more quickly, spend less

time in the hospital, and are more satisfied because they feel cared for as well as more hopeful and motivated. Families are satisfied with the personal care that their loved ones have received and tell the hospital administrator, who passes on the compliments to the physician, nursing staff, chaplain, and other health providers involved in the patients' care. Each of them feels good about their jobs. Patients are ill for a shorter time and return to the hospital and doctor less often, thus reducing the cost of medical care and reducing the time needed with the doctor on subsequent visits. Everybody wins!

Contrast this outcome to what happens in Drearyville in the "control" hospital without the educational intervention. In this hospital, spiritual care is not addressed. Because spiritual care is not a focus for any of the healthcare providers, the patient's spiritual needs are neglected. The unidentified needs continue to subtly and not-so-subtly influence the patient's medical condition and course of illness.

Because the patient is not improving and seems dissatisfied with the physician, the entire healthcare team, and the care plan, the physician uses more and more of the latest expensive technologies to diagnose why the patient isn't getting better. The rest of the team pulls away from the patient, assessing that the patient is "difficult." Of course, the patient continues to feel neglected, continues to struggle with unmet existential and spiritual needs, and ultimately loses hope and gives up. The patient, feeling hopeless and that no one cares, fails to comply with the medical plan. This affects rehabilitation, health outcomes, and subsequent rehospitalization and frequency of physician visits for failure to improve—due in part to unmet psychosocial and spiritual needs.

The entire healthcare team becomes frustrated with the patient and begins to see the patient as a "crock." They feel drained as a result of caring for this patient. Since nothing seems to be working, and because of poor communication, conflict ensues with the patient and the patient's family. The result: patient dissatisfaction, prolonged recovery, intense nursing care, frequent relapses, physician dissatisfaction and burnout, and use of expensive, high-tech, unnecessary diagnostic evaluation and extended treatment. Because of "bad outcomes" the patient's family sues the hospital and everyone involved in the care. Malpractice premiums go up, the physician moves to another state, and several nurses leave nursing. Nobody wins—except the lawyers!

A GLIMPSE INTO THE FUTURE

What might our healthcare system look like in ten years as a result of implementation of this educational intervention in just a few key medical centers? Although highly speculative and more than a bit optimistic, we would predict the following scenario. Let's return to Pleasantville and suppose that top administrators and influential health professionals (primarily those who are themselves spiritual and value the importance of spirituality) at four major medical centers advocate for educational programs for health professionals that train providers to take a spiritual history/assessment and respond to the spiritual needs revealed through that process.

As a result of such training, instead of 5 to 10 percent of health professionals addressing patients' spiritual needs, this proportion increases to 25 to 35 percent at these institutions. Health professionals who begin addressing patients' spiritual needs discover that patients deeply appreciate this, are more satisfied with their care, comply better because of greater trust, get better a little quicker, and use fewer expensive health services.

Hospital administrators soon discover that not only are patients more satisfied and less litigious, but also that the reputation of the hospital within the community improves, and there is less staff turnover in their hospitals (due to greater provider satisfaction, and to a reduction in malpractice rates because there are fewer lawsuits). This, of course, gives these hospitals a competitive advantage over other hospitals, resulting in more patients and more revenue.

Because of what appears to be happening in these leading academic healthcare systems, both NIH (given potential Medicare savings) and private insurance companies (for the same reason) start sponsoring research that examines the effects of addressing spiritual needs on provider-patient relationships, health outcomes, and need for health services. New research findings from these studies validate the benefits of addressing patients' (and providers') spiritual needs. This research is publicized in medical and hospital administration journals, and soon a wave of staff educational programs spreads across hospitals throughout the United States. Addressing patients' spiritual needs now becomes mainstream, healthcare costs drop, and both patient and provider satisfaction increase. Welcome to Pleasantville!

Is this possible? Is it a fanciful dream?

Let's end with the words of Antoine de Saint-Exupery:[2]

A rock pile ceases to be a rock pile the moment a single man contemplates it, bearing within him the image of a cathedral.

Let's dream on!

APPENDIX A

Religious Beliefs and Practices

In chapter 4, we mentioned the need for familiarity with different faith traditions. Following are summaries of the beliefs and practices of Judaism,
Christianity, Islam, and Eastern religious traditions:[1]

JEWISH BELIEFS AND PRACTICES AFFECTING HEALTHCARE

Observant Jews (Orthodox Judaism and some Conservative Jewish groups)

Birth: For observant Jews, babies are named by the father. Male children
are named 8 days after birth, when ritual circumcision is done. Circumcision
may be postponed if the infant is in poor health. Female babies are usually
named during the reading of the Holy Torah. Nurses need to be sensitive to the
wishes of the parents when caring for babies who have not yet been named.

Care of Women: A woman is considered to be in a ritual state of impurity
whenever blood is coming from her uterus, such as during menstrual periods
and after the birth of a child. During this time, her husband will not have physical contact with her. When this time is completed, she will bathe herself in a
pool called a mikvah. Nurses need to be aware of this practice and be sensitive
to the husband and wife because the husband will not touch his wife. He
cannot assist her in moving in the bed, so the nurse will have to do this.
An Orthodox Jewish man will not touch any women other than his wife,
daughters, and mother. Home healthcare workers need to be aware of these
practices.

Dietary rules: (1) Kosher dietary laws include the following: No mixing of
milk and meat at a meal; no consumption of food or any derivative thereof
from animals not slaughtered in accordance with Jewish law; use of separate

cooking utensils for milk and meat products; if a client requires milk and meat products for a meal, the dairy foods should be served first, followed later by the meat. (2) During Yom Kippur (Day of Atonement), a twenty-four-hour fast is required, but exceptions are made for those who cannot fast because of medical reasons. (3) During Passover, no leavened products are eaten. (4) May say benediction of thanksgiving before meals and grace at the end of the meal. Time and a quiet environment should be provided for this.

Sabbath: Observed from sunset Friday until sunset Saturday. Orthodox law prohibits riding in a car, smoking, turning lights on and off, handling money, and using television and telephone. Nurses need to be aware of this when caring for observant Jews at home and in the hospital. Medical or surgical treatments should be postponed if possible.

Death: Judaism defines death as occurring when respiration and circulation are irreversibly stopped and no movement is apparent. (1) Euthanasia is strictly forbidden by Orthodox Jews, who advocate the strict use of life-support measures. (2) Prior to death, Jewish faith indicates that visiting of the person by family and friends is a religious duty. The Torah and Psalms may be read and prayers recited. A witness needs to be present when a person prays for health so that if death occurs God will protect the family and the spirit will be committed to God. Extraneous talking and conversation about death are not encouraged unless initiated by the patient or visitors. In Judaism, the belief is that people should have someone with them when the soul leaves the body, so family and/or friends should be allowed to stay with patients. After death, the body should not be left alone until buried, usually within 24 hours. (3) When death occurs, the body should be untouched for 8 to 30 minutes. Medical personnel should not touch or wash the body but allow only an Orthodox person or the Jewish Burial Society to care for the body. Handling of a corpse on the Sabbath is forbidden to Jewish persons. If need be, the nursing staff may provide routine care of the body, wearing gloves. Water in the room should be emptied, and the family may request that mirrors be covered to symbolize that a death has occurred. (4) Orthodox Jews and some Conservative Jews do not approve of autopsies. If an autopsy must be done, all body parts must remain with the body. (5) For Orthodox Jews, the body must be buried within 24 hours. No flowers are permitted. A fetus must be buried. (6) A 7-day mourning period is required for the immediate family. They must stay at home except for Sabbath worship. (7) Organs or other body parts such as amputated limbs must be made available for burial for Orthodox Jews, since they believe that all of the body must be returned to earth.

Birth control and abortion: Artificial methods of birth control are not encouraged. Vasectomy is not allowed. Abortion may be performed only to save the mother's life.

Organ transplant: Donor organs generally are not permitted by Orthodox Jews but may be allowed with rabbinical consent.

Shaving: The beard is regarded as a mark of piety among observant Jews. For the very Orthodox, shaving should not be done with a razor but with scissors or an electric razor, since a blade should not contact the skin.

Head covering: Orthodox men wear skull caps at all times, and women cover their hair after marriage. Some Orthodox women wear wigs as a mark of piety. Conservative Jews cover their heads only during acts of worship and prayer.

Prayer: Praying directly to God, including a prayer of confession, is required for Orthodox Jews. Nurses should provide quiet time for prayer.

Reform Jews

Birth: Reform Jews may or may not adhere to the practices referred to for observant Jews. They favor ritual circumcision, but it is not imperative.

Care of women: Reform Jews do not observe the rules against touching.

Dietary rules: Reform Jews usually do not observe kosher dietary restrictions.

Sabbath: Usually worship in temples on Friday evenings. No strict rules.

Death: Advocate use of life support without heroic measures. Allow for cremation but suggest that ashes be buried in a Jewish cemetery.

Organ transplants: Donation or transplantation of organs allowed with permission of a rabbi.

Head coverings: Generally pray without wearing skull caps.

ROMAN CATHOLIC AND EASTERN ORTHODOX BELIEFS AND PRACTICES AFFECTING HEALTHCARE

Roman Catholic

Birth: Since Roman Catholics believe that unbaptized children are cut off from heaven, infant baptism is mandatory. For newborns with a grave prognosis, stillborns, and all aborted fetuses (unless evidence of tissue necrosis and prolonged death are present), emergency baptism is required. The nurse calls a priest to perform the baptism unless the death might occur before the priest arrives. In that case, anyone can baptize by pouring warm water on the infant's head and saying, "I baptize you in the name of the Father, of the Son, and of the Holy Spirit." All information about the baptism is recorded on the chart, and the priest and the family notified.

Holy Eucharist: For clients and healthcare givers who are to receive communion, abstinence from solid food and alcohol is required for 15 minutes (if possible) prior to reception of the consecrated wafer. Medicine, water, and non-alcoholic drinks are permitted at any time. If a client is in danger of health, the fast is waived since the reception of the Eucharist at this time is very important.

Anointing of the sick: The priest uses oil to anoint the forehead and hands and, if desired, the affected area. The rite may be performed on any who are ill and desire it. Persons receiving the sacrament seek complete healing, and strength to endure suffering. Prior to 1963, this sacrament was only given to persons at time of imminent death, so the nurse must be sensitive to the meaning this has for the client. If possible, the nurse calls before the client is unconscious but may also call when there is sudden death, since the sacrament may also be given shortly after death. The nurse records on the care plan that this sacrament has been administered.

Dietary habits: Obligatory fasting is excused during hospitalization. However, if there are no health restrictions, some Catholics may still observe the following guidelines: (1) Anyone 14 years or older must abstain from eating meat on Ash Wednesday and all Fridays during Lent. Some older Catholics may still abstain from meat on all Fridays of the year. (2) In addition to abstinence from meat, persons 21 to 59 years of age must limit themselves to one full meal and two light meals on Ash Wednesday and Good Friday. (3) Eastern Rite Catholics are stricter about fasting and fast more frequently than Western Rite Catholics, so it is important for the nurse to know if a client is Eastern or Western.

Death: Each Roman Catholic should participate in the anointing of the sick as well as the Eucharist and penance before death. The body should not be shrouded until these sacraments are performed. All body parts that retain human quality must be appropriately buried or cremated.

Birth control: Prohibited except for abstinence or natural family planning. Referral to a priest for questions about this can be of great help. Nurses can teach the techniques of natural family planning if they are familiar with them; otherwise, this should be referred to the physician or to a support group of the church that instructs couples in this method of birth control. Sterilization is prohibited unless there is an overriding medical reason.

Organ donation: Donation and transplantation of organs are acceptable as long as the donor is not harmed and is not deprived of life.

Religious objects: Rosary prayers are said using rosary beads. Medals bearing the images of saints, relics, statues, and scapulars are important objects that may be pinned to a hospital gown or pillow or be at the bedside. Extreme care should be taken not to lose these objects, since they have special meaning to the client.

Eastern Orthodox

Birth: The child must be baptized within 40 days after birth. If sprinkling or immersion into water is not possible, baptism is performed by moving the baby in the air in the sign of the cross. An ordained priest or a deacon must be notified for this.

Holy Eucharist: The priest is notified if the client desires this sacrament.

Anointing of the sick: The priest conducts this in the hospital room.

Dietary habits: Fasting from meat and dairy products is required on Wednesday and Friday during Lent and on other holy days. Hospital clients are exempt if fasting is detrimental to health.

Special days: Christmas is celebrated on January 7 and New Year's on January 14. This is important to the care of a client who is hospitalized on these days.

Death: Last rites are obligatory. This is handled by an ordained priest who is notified by the nurse while the client is conscious. The Russian Orthodox Church does not encourage autopsy or organ donation. Euthanasia, even for the terminally ill, is discouraged, as is cremation.

Birth control: This as well as abortion is not permitted.

VARIOUS PROTESTANT BELIEFS AND PRACTICES AFFECTING HEALTHCARE

Assemblies of God (Pentecostal)

Baptism: Water baptism by complete immersion is practiced when an individual has received Jesus Christ as savior and Lord based on Acts 2:38.

Holy Communion: Notify clergy if client desires.

Anointing of the sick: Members believe in divine healing through prayer and the laying on of hands. Clergy is notified if client or family desires this.

Dietary habits: Abstinence from alcohol, tobacco, and all illegal drugs is strongly encouraged.

Death: No special practices.

Other practices: Faith in God and in the healthcare providers is encouraged. Members pray for divine intervention in health matters. Nurses should encourage and allow time for prayer. Members may speak in "tongues" during prayer.

Baptist (over 27 different groups in the United States)

Baptism: Do not practice infant baptism.

Holy Communion: Clergy should be notified if the client desires.

Dietary habits: Total abstinence from alcohol is expected.

Death: No general service is provided, but the clergy does minister through counseling, prayer, and scripture as requested by the client or family, and the client is encouraged to believe in Jesus Christ as Savior and Lord.

Other practices: The Bible is held to be the word of God, so the nurse should either allow quiet time for Scripture reading or offer to read to the client.

Christian Church (Disciples of Christ)

Baptism: Do not practice infant baptism but have dedication service. Believers are baptized by immersion.

Holy Communion: Open communion is celebrated each Sunday and is a central part of worship services. The nurse notifies the clergy if the client desires it, or the clergy may suggest it.

Death: No special practices.

Other practices: Church elders as well as clergy may be notified to assist with meeting the client's spiritual needs.

Church of the Brethren

Baptism: Do not practice infant baptism but have dedication service.

Holy Communion: Usually received within church, but clergy will give it in the hospital when requested.

Anointing of the sick: Practiced for physical healing as well as spiritual uplift and held in high regard by the church. The clergy is notified if the client or family desire.

Death: The clergy is notified for counsel and prayer.

Church of the Nazarene

Baptism: Parents have the choice of baptism or dedication for their infant. Emphasis is on the believer's baptism, which is regarded as a symbol of the New Covenant in Jesus Christ.

Holy Communion: Pastor will administer if the client wishes.

Dietary habits: The use of alcohol and tobacco is forbidden.

Death: Cremation is permitted, and term stillborn infants are buried.

Other practices: Believe in divine healing but not to the exclusion of medical treatment. Clients may desire quiet time for prayer.

Episcopal (Anglican)

Baptism: Infant baptism is practiced and considered urgent if the infant is critically ill. The priest is notified to administer the sacrament. Lay persons may baptize in an emergency.

Holy Communion: The priest is notified if the client wishes to receive this sacrament.

Anointing of the sick: Priest may administer this rite when death is imminent, but it is not considered mandatory.

Dietary habits: Some clients may abstain from meat on Fridays. Others may fast before receiving the Eucharist, but fasting is not mandatory.

Death: No special practices.

Other practices: Confession of sins to a priest is optional; if the client desires this, the clergy should be notified.

Lutheran (10 Different Branches)

Baptism: Baptize only living infants any time, but usually 6 to 8 weeks after birth. Adults are baptized, and modes of baptism as appropriate include sprinkling, pouring, or immersion.

Holy Communion: Notify the clergy if the client desires this sacrament. Clergy may also inquire about the client's desire.

Anointing of the sick: The client may request an anointing and blessing from the minister when the prognosis is poor.

Death: A service of Commendation of the Dying is used at the client's or family's request.

Mennonite (12 Different Groups)

Baptism: No infant baptism, but the child may be dedicated if requested by the parents.

Holy Communion: Served twice a year, with foot washing as part of the ceremony.

Dietary habits: Abstinence from alcohol is urged for all.

Death: Prayer is important at time of crisis, so contacting a minister is important.

Other practices: Women may wear head coverings during hospitalization. Anointing with oil is administered in harmony with James 5:14 when requested.

Methodist (Over 20 Different Groups)

Baptism: Notify the clergy if the patient desires baptism for a sick infant.

Holy Communion: Notify the clergy if a client requests it prior to surgery or another health crisis.

Anointing of the sick: If requested, the clergy will come to pray and sprinkle the client with olive oil.

Death: Scripture reading and prayer are important at this time.

Other practices: Donation of one's body or part of the body at death is encouraged.

Presbyterian (10 Different Groups)

Baptism: Infant baptism is practiced by pouring or sprinkling. Immersion is also practiced at times for adults.

Holy Communion: Given when appropriate and convenient, at the hospitalized client's request.

Death: Notify a local pastor or elder for prayer and Scripture reading if desired by the family or client.

Quaker (Friends)

Baptism and Holy Communion: Since Friends have no creed there is a diversity of personal beliefs, one of which is that outward sacraments are usually not necessary since there is the ministry of the Spirit inwardly in such areas such as baptism and communion. A few Friends baptize with water.

Death: Believe that the present life is part of God's kingdom and generally have no ceremony as a rite of passage from this life to the next. Personal beliefs and wishes need to be ascertained, and the nurse can then act on the client's wishes.

Other practices: The name of the Quaker infant is recorded in official record books at the local meeting.

Salvation Army

Baptism: No particular ceremony, but they do have an Infant Dedication ceremony.

Holy Communion: No particular ceremony.

Death: Notify the local officer in charge of the Army Corps for any soldier (member) who needs assistance.

Other practices: The Bible is seen as the only rule for one's faith, so the Scriptures should be made available to a client. The Army has many of its own social welfare centers, with hospitals and homes where unwed mothers are cared for and outpatient services provided. No medical or surgical procedures are opposed, except for abortion on demand.

Seventh-Day Adventist

Baptism: No infant baptism is practiced, but have dedication services.

Holy Communion: Although this is not required of hospitalized clients, the clergy is notified if the client desires.

Anointing of the sick: The clergy are contacted for prayer and anointing with oil.

Dietary habits: Since the body is viewed as the temple of the Holy Spirit, healthy living is essential. Therefore the use of alcohol, tobacco, coffee, and tea and the promiscuous use of drugs are prohibited. Some are vegetarians, and most avoid pork.

Special days: The Sabbath is observed on Saturday.

Death: No special procedures.

Other related practices: Use of hypnotism is opposed by some. Persons of homosexual or lesbian orientation are ministered to in the hope of correction of these practices, which are believed to be wrong. A Bible should always be available for Scripture reading.

United Church of Christ

Baptism: Practice infant and adult baptism. Three modes are used as appropriate: pouring, sprinkling, and immersion.

Holy Communion: Clergy is notified if the client desires to receive this sacrament.

Death: If the client desires counsel or prayer, notify the clergy.

ISLAMIC AND MUSLIM BELIEFS AND PRACTICES AFFECTING HEALTHCARE

Islam

Birth: A baby is bathed immediately after birth, before giving it to the mother. The father (or the mother if the father is not available) then whispers the call to prayer in the child's ears so that the first sounds it hears are about the Muslim faith. Circumcision is culturally recommended before puberty. A baby born prematurely but at least 130 days gestation is given the same treatment as any other infant.

Dietary habits: No pork is allowed, nor alcoholic beverages. All halal (permissible) meat must be blessed and killed in a certain way. This is called zabihah (correctly slaughtered).

Death: Prior to death, family members ask to be present so that they can read the Koran and pray with the client. An Imam may come if requested by the client or family but is not required. Clients must face Mecca and confess their sins and beg forgiveness in the presence of their family. If the family is unavailable, any practicing Muslim can provide support to the client. After death, Muslims prefer that the family wash, prepare, and place the body in a position facing Mecca. If necessary, the healthcare providers may perform these procedures as long as they wear gloves. Burial is performed as soon as possible. Cremation is forbidden. Autopsy is also prohibited except for legal reasons, and then no body part is to be removed. Donation of body parts or organs is not allowed, since according to culturally developed law persons do not own their own body.

Abortion and birth control: Abortion is forbidden, and many conservative Muslims do not encourage the use of contraceptives since this interferes with God's purpose. Others feel that a woman should only have as many children as her husband can afford. Contraception is permitted by Islamic law.

Personal devotions: At prayer time, washing is required, even by those who are sick. A client on bed rest may require assistance with this task before prayer. Provision of privacy is important for prayer.

Religious objects: The Koran must not be touched by anyone ritually unclean, and nothing should be placed on top of it. Some Muslims wear taviz, a black string on which words of the Koran are attached. These should not be removed and must remain dry. Certain items of jewelry such as bangles may have religious significance and should not be removed unnecessarily.

Care of women: Since women are not allowed to sign consent forms or make a decision regarding family planning, the husband needs to be present. Women are very modest and frequently wear clothes that cover all of the body. During a medical examination, the woman's modesty should be respected as much as possible. Muslim women prefer female doctors. For 40 days after giving birth and also during menstruation, a woman is exempt from prayer since this is a time of cleansing for her.

American Muslim Mission

Baptism: No baptism is practiced.

Dietary habits: In addition to refusing pork, many will not eat traditional Southern American foods such as corn bread and collard greens.

Death: The family is contacted before any care of the deceased is performed. There are special procedures for washing and shrouding the body.

Other practices: Quiet time is necessary to permit prayer. Members are encouraged to use black physicians for health care. Since these clients do not smoke, their request for a nonsmoking roommate should be honored.

CHRISTIAN SCIENCE, JEHOVAH'S WITNESSES,
THE CHURCH OF JESUS CHRIST OF LATTER-DAY SAINTS,
UNITARIAN UNIVERSALIST, AND UNIFICATION CHURCH BELIEFS
AND PRACTICES AFFECTING HEALTHCARE

Christian Science

Birth: Use physician or nurse midwife during childbirth. No baptism ceremony.

Dietary habits: Since alcohol and tobacco are considered drugs, they are not used. Coffee and tea are often declined.

Other practices: Do not normally seek medical care, since they approach health care in a different, primarily spiritual, framework. They commonly utilize the services of a surgeon to set a bone but decline drugs and, in general, other medical or surgical procedures. Hypnotism and psychotherapy are also declined. Family planning is left to the family. They seek exemption from vaccinations but obey legal requirements. Report infectious diseases and obey public health quarantines. Nonmedical care facilities are maintained for those needing nursing assistance in the course of a healing. *The Christian Science Journal* lists available Christian Science nurses. When a Christian Science believer is in the hospital, the nurse should allow and encourage time for prayer and study. Clients may request that a Christian Science practitioner be notified to come.

Jehovah's Witnesses

Baptism: No infant baptism is practiced. Baptism by complete immersion of adults is done as a symbol of dedication to Jehovah, since Jesus was baptized.

Dietary habits: Use of alcohol and tobacco is discouraged, since these harm the physical body.

Death: Autopsy is a private matter to be decided by the persons involved. Burial and cremation are acceptable.

Birth control and abortion: Use of birth control is a personal decision. Abortion is opposed based on Exodus 21:22–23.

Organ transplants: Use of organ transplant is a private decision and if used must be cleansed with a nonblood solution.

Blood transfusions: Blood transfusions violate God's laws and are therefore not allowed. Clients do respect physicians and will accept alternatives to blood transfusions. These might include the use of nonblood plasma expanders, careful surgical techniques to decrease blood loss, use of autologous transfusions, and auto transfusion through use of a heart–lung machine. Nurses should check unconscious clients for medic alert cards that state that the person does not want a transfusion. Since Jehovah's Witnesses are prepared to die rather than break God's law, nurses need to be sensitive to the spiritual as well as the physical needs of the client.

The Church of Jesus Christ of Latter-Day Saints

Baptism: If a child over the age of eight is very ill, whether baptized or unbaptized, a member of the church's priesthood should be called.

Holy Communion: A hospitalized client may desire to have a member of the church priesthood administer this sacrament.

Anointing of the sick: Mormons frequently are anointed and given a blessing before going to the hospital and after admission by laying on of hands.

Dietary habits: Abstinence from the use of tobacco; beverages with caffeine such as cola, coffee, and tea; alcohol and other substances considered injurious. Mormons eat meat but encourage the intake of fruits, grains, and herbs.

Death: Prefer burial of the body. A church elder should be notified to assist the family. If need be, the elder will assist the funeral director in dressing the body in special clothes and will give other help as needed.

Birth control and abortion: Abortion is opposed except when the health of the mother is in danger. Only natural means of birth control are recommended. Artificial means can be used when the health of the woman is at stake (including emotional health).

Personal care: Cleanliness is very important to Mormons. A sacred undergarment may be worn at all times by Mormons and should only be removed in emergency situations.

Other practices: Allowing quiet time for prayer and the reading of the sacred writings is important. The church maintains a welfare system to help those in need. Families are of great importance, so visiting should be encouraged.

Unitarian Universalist Association

Baptism: Infant baptism is unnecessary and if used at all is without trinitarian formula. Usually dedicate their children.

Death: Cremation is often preferred to burial.

Other practices: Use of birth control is advocated as part of responsible parenting. Strong support for a woman's right to choice regarding abortion is maintained. Unitarian Universalists advocate donation of body parts for research and transplants.

Unification Church

Baptism: No baptism.

Special days: Sunday mornings are used to honor Reverend and Mrs. Moon as the true parents, and members get up at 5:00 A.M., bow before a picture of the Moons three times, and vow to do what is needed to help the Reverend accomplish his mission on earth.

Death: Believe that after death one's place of destiny will depend on his or her spirit's quality of life and goodness while on earth. In the afterlife, one will have the same aspirations and feelings as before death. Hell is not a concern, since it will not be a place as heaven grows in size. Persons who leave the Unification Church are warned that Satan may try to possess them.

Other practices: All marriages must be solemnized by Reverend Moon in order to be part of the perfect family and have salvation. The church supplies its faithful members with life's necessities. Members may use occult practices to have spiritual and psychic experiences.

(Permission from V. B. Carson [1989], *Spiritual Dimensions of Nursing Practice,* W. B. Saunders Company, 80–81, 85–86, 90–92, 95–96, 100–102.)

NON-WESTERN RELIGIOUS TRADITIONS BELIEFS AND PRACTICES AFFECTING HEALTHCARE

And here are summaries of the beliefs and practices of the non-Western religious traditions:[2]

Confucianism

Background. Confucianism is a transformation of ancient and traditional Chinese religious beliefs and practices centering on ethical and social dimensions and effects. This tradition was founded by K'ung Fu-tzu in the sixth century B.C.E., continuing and developing into a philosophical as well as a bureaucratic system until modern times in China, Korea, Japan, and Vietnam. The most important principles are filial piety and proper conduct. The former is the support of and obedience to parents, care of oneself and one's offspring, and reverence of ancestors. Some practical effects of the Confucian system are that care of the elderly is a family responsibility, and it is the male offspring's responsibility to ensure this, since women live with the husband's family.

Special days. Days for honoring ancestors on the lunar calendar include the third day of the third month, fifteenth day of the seventh month, and first day of the tenth month. Food, incense and prayers, and visits to tidy graves are the observances.

Writings. Five classics—the Book of Changes, the Book of Documents, the Book of Poetry, the Records of Rites, and the Spring and Autumn Annals—plus the Four Books, including the writings of the four philosophers, Kongzi (Confucius), the Analects, Lunyu and his disciple Zeng Shen, the Great Learning Daxue, the Doctrine of the Mean, and the Book of Mengzi. These are used for traditional Chinese education.

Buddhism

Background. Buddhism is a religion of understanding rather than of belief. It began in India in the sixth century B.C.E. Today there are more than 261 million Buddhists in the world, with much diversity. The main movements are the Theravada of Southern India, who follow the original form of Buddhism, and the Mahayan, who tend to be more liberal and emphasize enlightenment of the general public in the context of modern times. Buddhists see life as an inevitable process of birth, aging, illness, and death and believe that liberation from suffering occurs through the doctrine of the "Middle Way" (that is, attainment of Enlightenment Nirvana). Buddhists may also practice ancestor worship, Confucianism, Shintoism, and/or Taoism.

Holy days. No special day for prayer; most Buddhists celebrate Full Moon Day in May, as well as Buddha's birth, enlightenment, and passing.

Diet. May be vegan, lacto-ovo-vegetarian, or semivegetarian, depending on the form of Buddhism and on the part of the country of origin.

Prayers. Usually five times daily.

Sacred writings. The Tripitaka contains the sermons, precepts, and commentaries of Buddha.

Terminal illness/death. May wish a quiet place for meditation. "Last Rites" performed by Buddhist monk; prefer cremation.

Hinduism

Background. The Hindu deity is Brahman, Om or Aum, whose Supreme Being is manifested through lesser gods, including Vishnu and Shiva (Siva).

There are several divisions within the Hindu faith, giving rise to differences in daily religious practices, rituals, and ceremonies. Hinduism is a religion and a way of life with its origins before written history. It is followed by 80 percent of the population in India. Hindus believe that inequalities of birth or mental and physical disabilities are the result of deeds during past lives. Individuals are rewarded by being born into a better or worse situation according to their actions or karma in the previous life. The focus of the Hindu's life is the performance of one's duty, the honest attainment of wealth, the pursuit of unselfish desires, and the achievement of self-realization. Salvation is attained through the paths of knowledge, action, and devotion, with a synthesis of all three as the ideal. With love and devotion, an individual can achieve self-realization, but most important is the love of God.

Holy days. Dates follow the lunar calendar and tend to be observed locally or regionally. Holy days are observed with fasting, prayer, and feasting.

Diet. May be unrestricted or vegan to semivegetarian, depending upon the form of Hinduism and the part of the country of origin. May prefer to eat only what is brought in by family; may prefer disposable dishes and cutlery; no alcohol or tobacco products; nonvegetarians may refuse beef and pork and their products; may eat only with right hand.

Fasting. Some Hindus fast several times a week from sunrise to sunset; fasting may take different forms, such as taking one meal per day, abstaining from a particular food, or abstaining from all food and liquids for a designated time.

Prayer. Hindus usually pray and meditate twice daily—privacy is required; may wish to have holy books and prayer beads; many older people withdraw from the world to spend their lives in prayer and meditation.

Clothing/modesty. Women cover upper arms, breasts, and legs. Men cover from waist to knees. Both prefer their own pants or shorts with hospital gowns (hospital gowns are considered indecent); same-sex providers are preferred.

Visitors. Staying with the ill patient is important to both the patient and family; it is important to explain visiting hours and to be flexible with them if possible.

Scriptures. Four Vedas, the Upanishads, and the Epics—the Mahabharata (which includes the Bhagavad-Gita) and the Ramayana—are all in Sanskrit.

Religious symbols. Some women wear a thread around the neck and a red mark on the forehead, and these should not be removed. Some men wear a thread around the right shoulder or around the waist or arm and prayer beads.

Local religious leader. Guru—guide and teacher in the temple *(mandir).*

Religious rites: Samskaras are the rites by which a Hindu becomes a full member of the socioreligious community; associated with birth, naming of child, puberty, and death.

Terminal illness/death. Family members expect to care for patients who are ill and dying and will read aloud, sing, and pray. Hindus usually wish to die at home, preferably on the floor to be closer to Mother Earth. Open expression of grief is usual after a death. If death occurs in hospital, family members usually prepare the body. If family members are not available, staff should wear disposable gloves, close the eyes, and straighten the limbs. A plain sheet should wrap the body. The body should not be washed by the staff. Religious objects remain with the body. Cremation is usual.

Cleanliness. Cleanliness includes preferably a daily shower, washing with running water to purify oneself before prayers, before and after meals, and after using the bathroom. The right hand is considered clean and the left hand unclean.

Sikhism

Background. Sikhism is a monotheistic religion found by Guru Nanak (1469–1539) in Northern India. The word *Sikh* means a learner or disciple. Sikhs are encouraged to live by honest work as a householder, to share success with the less fortunate, and always to be grateful to the Almighty. The conduct of life for the Sikh is knowledge, devotion, and action, guided by those who have gone before. After baptism, men are called Singh and women are called Kaur.

Holy days. Celebrate important events in the early history of Sikhism following the lunar calendar; Baisakhi or New Year's, commemoration of Guru Nanak's birth date.

Diet. Individual choice, although many are lacto-ovo-vegetarian or semi-vegetarian; usually no beef or pork. No tobacco products or intoxicants are permitted.

Fasting. Not a usual practice.

Prayers. Privacy is preferred; recitation morning and evening.

Clothing/modesty. Women cover upper arms, breasts, and legs; men cover from waist to knees; both prefer their own or facility pants with hospital gowns over them; same-sex caregivers are important to both sexes.

Scriptures. Holy book is the Guru Granth Sahib (the writings of Guru Nanak and later gurus). Rehat Maryada describes their code of conduct and provides guidelines for daily living.

Religious symbols: Kesh, uncut hair—Sikhs may refuse to have any body hair cut (including for attachment of EKG electrodes); *kangha*, comb; *Kara*, steel bracelet, never removed from right wrist, symbolizes strength and unity; *kirpan*, symbolic dagger, symbolizes authority; *kachha*, special undershorts for both sexes, symbolizes freedom; turban for men, which is worn twenty-four hours a day. The removal of any Sikh symbol should only be done after consultation with the patient.

Local religious leader: Giani, a learned man, not a holy man, who serves in the temple *(Gurdwara)*.

Terminal illness/death. Prayers and hymns may be recited by the patient or read aloud by family members for comfort. Religious symbols stay with the patient. After death, close eyes and mouth; do not cut nails, hair, or beard; cover with plain white sheet. Cremation is preferred.

Cleanliness. Prefer to wash with running water before and after eating and before prayers; prefer showers to baths; right hand is considered clean and left hand unclean.

Taoism

Background. Taoism is an ancient Chinese way of life that dates back to the philosopher Lao-Tze, who lived 500 B.C.E. Taoism advocates that one should let events run their natural course, keep a tranquil mind, and live as close to nature as possible. Simplicity and humility lead the way to personal harmony. Taoism is often practiced with Confucianism and/or Buddhism.

Special days. According to the lunar calendar; for honoring ancestors; New Year's Day, Dragon Boat Festival; and deity birthdays.

Sacred writings. Many and vast; main text is Tao Te Ching, attributed to Lao Tzu.

Addendum. Taoist masters may perform exorcism of malevolent spirits causing illness or misfortune.

(Permission from K. J. Griffith (1996), *The Religious Aspects of Nursing Care*, Box 72072, 4479 W. Tenth Avenue, Vancouver, B.C., Canada V6R 4P2.)

Spiritual Assessment Resources

In addition to the information presented in chapter 5 concerning ways to obtain a spiritual history, a number of additional spiritual assessment tools are available. Although most of these assessments are developed by physicians, they could easily be used by other healthcare professionals. We include a few for your consideration.

THE FICA

The FICA was developed by Dr. Christina Puchalski, founder and director of the George Washington Institute for Spirituality and Health.[1] This assessment tool is brief and patient centered, and it is easy to remember using the income-tax mnemonic FICA.

F—Faith and Belief. Do you consider yourself spiritual or religious? Or do you have spiritual beliefs that help you cope with stress? If the patient responds "No," the healthcare provider might ask, "What gives your life meaning?" Sometimes patients respond with answers such as family, career, or nature.

I—Importance. What importance does your faith or belief have in your life? Have your beliefs influenced how you take care of yourself in this illness? What role do your beliefs play in regaining your health?

C—Community. Are you part of a spiritual or religious community? Is this of support to you, and if so, how? Is there a group of people you really love or who are important to you? Communities such as churches, temples, and mosques, or a group of like-minded friends can serve as strong support systems for some patients.

A—Apply. How do your religious and spiritual beliefs apply to your health?

A—Address. How might we address your spiritual needs?

BRIEF SPIRITUAL HISTORY

This brief spiritual history was developed by Dr. Harold G. Koenig.[2]

1. Do your religious or spiritual beliefs provide comfort and support, or do they cause stress?

2. How would these beliefs influence your medical decisions if you became really sick?

3. Do you have any beliefs that might interfere or conflict with your medical care?

4. Are you a member of a religious or spiritual community, and is it supportive?

5. Do you have any spiritual needs that someone should address?

MATTHEWS SPIRITUAL HISTORY

Dr. D. A. Matthews, an associate professor at Georgetown University, offers three questions for physicians to ask as part of their initial interview.[3]

1. Is religion or spirituality important to you?

2. Do your religious or spiritual beliefs influence the way you think about your medical problems and the way you think about your health?

3. Would you like me to address your spiritual beliefs and practices with you?

THE SPIRITUAL HISTORY

Developed by Todd Maugans, the SPIRITual History is a comprehensive assessment and takes more time to administer.[4] It might be quite useful in long-term care and homecare, where the time spent with patients is longer and the duration of care is extended.

Spiritual Belief System. What is your formal religious affiliation? Name or describe your spiritual belief system.

Personal Spirituality. Describe the beliefs and practices of your spiritual belief system that you personally accept. Describe the beliefs and practices that you do not accept. Do you accept or believe (fill in with a specific tenet or practice)? What does your spirituality/religion mean to you? What is the importance of your spirituality/religion in your daily life?

Integration within a Spiritual Community. Do you belong to any spiritual or religious group or community? What is your position or role? What importance does this group have to you? Is it a source of support? In what ways? Does or could this group provide help in dealing with health issues?

Ritualized Practices and Restrictions. Are there specific practices that you carry out as part of your religion/spirituality (e.g., prayer or meditation)? Are there certain lifestyle activities or practices that your religion/spirituality encourages or forbids? Do you comply? What significance do these practices and restrictions have to you? Are there specific elements of medical care that you forbid on religious/spiritual grounds?

Implications for Medical Care. What aspects of your religion/spirituality would you like me to keep in mind as I care for you? Would you like to discuss the religious or spiritual implications of health care? What knowledge or understanding of spiritual issues would strengthen our relationship as physician/nurse and patient?

Terminal Events Planning. As we plan for your care near the end of life, what impact does your faith have on your decisions? Are there particular aspects of care that you wish to forego or have withheld because of your faith?

THE HOPE ASSESSMENT TOOL

This spiritual assessment tool, developed by Gowri Anandarajah and Ellen Hight from Brown University, uses the mnemonic HOPE.[5] The tool is brief, patient centered, and easy to remember, and it provides valuable information.

H: Sources of Hope, Meaning, Comfort, Strength, Peace, Love, and Connection. What are your sources of hope, strength, comfort, and peace? What do you hold onto during difficult times? What sustains you and keeps you going?

O: Organized Religion. Are you part of a religious or spiritual community? Does it help you? How? What aspects of your religion are helpful and not so helpful to you?

P: Personal Spirituality and Practices. Do you have any personal spiritual beliefs that are independent of organized religion? What aspect of your spirituality or spiritual practices do you find most helpful to you personally?

E: Effects on Medical Care and End-of-Life Issues. Has being sick affected your ability to do things that usually help you spiritually? As a (nurse, doctor, etc.), is there anything that I can do to help you access resources that usually help you? Are there any specific practices or restrictions I should know about in providing your care?

THE ACP SPIRITUAL HISTORY

The ACP Spiritual History assessment tool was developed by a consensus panel of American College of Physicians and American Society of Internal Medicine.[6] It suggests four simple questions be asked of patients with serious medical illness. The instrument is brief, patient centered, and easy to remember.

1. Is faith (religion, spirituality) important to you in this illness?
2. Has faith been important to you at other times in your life?
3. Do you have someone to talk to about religious matters?
4. Would you like to explore religious matters with someone?

GERONTOLOGIC PASTORAL CARE INSTITUTE SPIRITUAL LIFE REVIEW AND NEEDS ASSESSMENT

The Gerontologic Pastoral Care Institute Spiritual Life Review and Needs Assessment was designed for the elderly; it has a Christian flavor but could be adapted to other faith traditions. It is a long and comprehensive tool, probably most appropriately used in its complete form by the chaplain. It could, however, be adapted to individual patient situations and has great applicability to long-term care, hospice care, and homecare.

Personal Information

Name _____

Address _____

Phone _____

Initial observation: Individual is

_____ alert and oriented _____ alert and disoriented

_____ unable to communicate

Religious affiliation _____

Level of congregational activity prior to admission:

_____ active _____ inactive

Desires visits from parish clergy and/or laypersons: _____ yes _____ no

If membership is with a congregation outside the geographic area, should that congregation be notified? _____ no _____ yes

Name & Address of Congregation: _____

_____

Desire for religious participation:

_____ Attend services _____ Bible reading and/or study

_____ Chaplain visits _____ Communion _____ Confession

_____ Hymn singing _____ Prayer _____ Other (explain):

Ability to attend religious activities:

_____ needs reminders _____ can transport self _____ needs escort

Religious Beliefs and Perceptions

Image of Jesus: _____ a loving, supportive friend
_____ distant, a person in Bible stories
_____ uncertain about an image of Jesus

Image of God: _____ loving, forgiving, and supportive
_____ punitive and angry _____ withdrawn, not present
_____ uncertain about an image of God

Suffering is: _____ punishment for sins _____ meaningless
_____ an inevitable part of life that allows for growth

Salvation is: _____ assured _____ denied _____ not understood

Strength and courage received from
_____ God _____ Jesus _____ family _____ self _____ friends _____ staff

Favorite hymns:_____

Favorite Scriptures:_____

Important Spiritual Experiences

I'm going to list some activities that may relate to your spiritual life. Tell me how important they are to you now:

3 = Important; 2 = neutral; 1 = not important.
_____ spending time thinking, meditating, or praying
_____ enjoying beauty: art, nature, music, etc.
_____ learning new things about your religion
_____ attending worship services
_____ reflecting on the meaning of your life
_____ sharing your spiritual life with others

Are there other important spiritual experiences you'd like to tell me about?

Are there important aspects of your spiritual life that you feel you're missing now?

Spiritual Life Review

1. Tell me a little about yourself and your childhood . . .
   a. How was your home heated?_____

b. Where was the center of warmth in your home? _____

c. Who was the person of warmth in your home? _____

d. When, if ever, did God become a person of warmth to you?

_____

2. Tell me about your experiences in churches through your life, beginning when you were a child and on through adulthood. _____

_____

3. What were some of the most positive experiences in your life?

_____

4. What are some of the sad experiences you've had? How did you cope with them? _____

_____

5. Who are the people important in your life now? How do they care for you? _____

_____

6. What do you think God is asking of you now? _____

_____

7. What are you asking of God now? _____

_____

Requests for the Time of Dying

_____ Music   _____ Clergy Present   _____ Family Present

_____ Last Rites   _____ Rosary   _____ The Sacrament

_____ Reading of Scripture (which passages?)   _____ Other (explain)

Pastoral evaluation and plans: _____

_____

Signs of spiritual strength: _____

_____

Signs of spiritual distress: _____

_____

Recommendations for pastoral care: _____

_____

Completed by_____Date:_____

Used with permission of The Center for Aging, Religion, and Spirituality, Luther Seminary, 2481 Como Avenue, St. Paul, MN 55108-1496. 651-641-1496, e-mail: Cars@luthersem.edu

Many thanks to Cheryl Hovland, parish nurse in Pelican Rapids, Minnesota, for sharing this resource with us. Cheryl can be reached at cherylhovland2@meritcare.com.

NURSING EDUCATION RESOURCES

Videos. Eight videos with accompanying facilitator's guides provide an excellent teaching tool regarding the nature of spirituality, conducting a spiritual assessment, and providing spiritual care across different clinical scenarios.

In the video dealing with spiritual assessment, for instance, three different people are interviewed: a very devout Christian, active in his church, with a clear sense of Christian spirituality; a middle-aged woman with a loose sense of spirituality who draws her beliefs from a wide variety of spiritual worldviews, including New Age thinking and Eastern as well as smatterings of Christian beliefs; and a young woman diagnosed with AIDS who struggles with the basic notion of whether God exists.

The assessments are conducted using the questions provided in chapter 5 (see pages 95–98).

These video resources were developed for nursing students, nurses, and other health professionals. Their titles follow:

Spirituality
Nurses and Spiritual Care
Spiritual Assessment
Spirituality in Palliative Care
Spiritual Care in Gerontological Nursing
Spiritual Care and Life Threatening Illness
Spirituality in Mental Health Care
Spiritual Care and Chronic Health Problems

The videos were developed by and are available for $130.00 each plus $10.00 shipping and handling from:

Doreen Westera, MScN, M.Ed.
Associate Professor
School of Nursing
Memorial University of Newfoundland
St. John's, NL Canada A1B 3V6
(709) 777-7259; fax (709) 777-7037; dwestera@mun.ca

SOCIAL WORK EDUCATIONAL RESOURCES

Publications. There are many text resources available to social workers interested in learning more about spirituality. The following is by no means an exhaustive listing:

Bullis, R. (1996), *Spirituality in Social Work Practice* (Washington, D.C.: Taylor and Francis).

Canda, E. R. (1988), "Spirituality, Religious Diversity, and Social Work Practice," *Social Case Work: The Journal of Contemporary Social Work*, Family Service America, 238–247.

Canda, E. R. (1998), *Spirituality in Social Work: New Directions* (New York: Haworth Pastoral Press).

Canda, E. R., and Fuhrman, L. D. (1999), *Spiritual Diversity in Social Work Practice: The Heart of Helping* (New York: Free Press).

Loewenberg, F. M. (1988), *Religion and Social Work Practice in Contemporary American Society* (New York: Columbia University Press).

Parrott, L. (2002), *Social Work and Social Care*, 2nd ed. (London: Routledge).

APPENDIX C

Resources for Spiritual Support and Nurture

In chapter 6 and chapter 9, we mentioned the value of journaling. We indicated that it is not only an excellent spiritual intervention for our patients, with the potential for improving their physical well-being, but that it is also an excellent strategy for each of us to examine our spirituality, feed our spirits, and remain reflective and focused on not only the "why" of our existence but also the "why" of our practice. Here are some suggested approaches to journaling.

REFLECTION: SELF-AWARENESS AND SPIRITUAL DEVELOPMENT

The purpose of this exercise is to help you reflect on the spiritual part of yourself and identify experiences that have shaped and contributed to your spiritual development.[1] The more we grow in self-awareness, the better we will be able to understand the spiritual development of our patients.

Reflect on the following questions and write what comes to your mind. Remember that this is for you. Don't be concerned with grammar, neatness, or sentence structure. The purpose is for you to look honestly at yourself. Be as open and honest as possible with your thoughts and feelings. Remember that your feelings cannot be judged, nor can your personal spiritual journey.

• Describe some event in your life that has contributed to your spiritual development. This may be a specific event, such as a traumatic or very happy experience. This event may have occurred in your family life, in your faith community, with a friend, with a peer at work, or with a patient for whom you provided care.

• Explain how this event changed you spiritually. What were some of your feelings? Responses? What did this event mean to you?

• If your reflection reveals difficult memories, what sustained you during these times?

• What role did your spirituality play in this experience?

• How would you describe where you are in your own spiritual development? Do you have a clear sense of who God is? Who you are? What your purpose is in this life? Or are you unsure of God and your relationship to God? Do you feel lost and disconnected, with a lack of purpose?

• How does your spirituality influence your family life, your relationships with friends, your work as a healthcare provider?

• Have you been drawn into a personally meaningful relationship with a supreme being or higher power?

• What events led you to establish this relationship?

You may wish to share this with a friend who is spiritually mature and who may help you gain some insight into yourself. Dialogue with a like-minded spiritual person is valuable in helping us to gain depth and understanding in our spiritual perspectives.

SELF REFLECTION: GETTING TO KNOW
YOUR SPIRITUAL SELF

Write in "free style" the feelings associated with your spiritual self. Find a quiet space and spend some time trying to get in touch with your self, with the very center of your being. Sit quietly and let go of your distractions. Copy the questions into your journal. Answer each of the questions using as much space as you require. Then, through poetry, song, music, art, or journaling allow your thoughts and feelings to flow. (A helpful hint in journaling is to address each of the questions by writing down all your thoughts and feelings until you have no more. If you draw or use an art form, provide a brief summary explaining the abstractions, colors, images, and feelings and how they reflect your spiritual self.)

• Who are you? (Write down your thoughts and feelings until you have no more.)

• How do you respond when you think about the possibility that your life could end tomorrow? Now who are you?

• What brings you to the very center of your being, where you cannot identify yourself according to your possessions, your accomplishments, your work, or who you're related to? *Who are you?*

• What gives meaning to your life?

• Who would you be if you could not do anything for yourself, or communicate with others as you do now?

WRITING YOUR SPIRITUAL AUTOBIOGRAPHY

Each of us has a spiritual story worth telling—not so much for the benefit of others, but for our own growth and enrichment.[2] As you consider your own spiritual autobiography, keep in mind that the goal is not to write a spiritual classic with enduring value. Writing your spiritual autobiography becomes a prayer, a form of spiritual discipline. It is private—something between you and God. Write what you really believe, not what you think you should believe. This autobiography should reflect an honest and humble appraisal of your actual beliefs as well as your challenges, struggles, and doubts.

Why undertake such a discipline? What is the value of this undertaking? First, the autobiography becomes a tool for personal accountability. If you are matching actions with your stated beliefs, then that will jump out at you; likewise, if you are giving only lip service and no action to what you say you believe, that also becomes apparent. Second, the spiritual autobiography is a way of connecting to and deepening a sense of community. As you write, you will naturally include experiences with others that influenced and shaped your spiritual journey. The autobiography will be as much a story about others in your life as your own story.

The tool for constructing the spiritual autobiography is the personal journal. Remember that the journal is intended to be a place of spiritual growth and exploration. It is a private place, a sanctuary within, where you can retreat for quiet reflection, for growth, and for shedding some tears.

How do you begin? How do you organize your spiritual autobiography? Consider beginning with a spiritual genealogy. Tell the story of faith (or lack thereof) of your parents, and their parents, and of earlier generations. This gives you insight into early influences and traditions that have shaped your journey.

You might want to generate a list of those people who have influenced your spiritual journey. Some of these persons may have been sources of inspiration; others may have been sources of pain. Your list may also include people you have never met but who have influenced you through their writings, their contributions, their lives.

You might also want to approach your spiritual autobiography in a chronological manner, beginning with early memories of spiritual experiences and ending with a summary of where you see yourself today. Reviewing such a chronology may reveal patterns and themes that have repeated through your life. You may better recognize the hand of God in your life. The lasting impact of both positive and negative events becomes apparent, as well as how your developmental stages affected your spirituality or vice versa. For instance, how did your adolescence affect your spirituality? This chronology can allow you to evaluate whether you have spiritually matured or whether you got "stuck" at a particular development stage.

Last, you can approach your spiritual autobiography by exploring different themes or issues. Questions such as the following could guide this exploration:

- What has been your experience with prayer? With unanswered prayer?
- How has your image of God changed over time?
- What types of suffering have you faced? How have these experiences of suffering affected your relationship with God? Have you ever been angry with God?
- How have loving relationships played a part in your spiritual journey?
- What role has doubt played in your spiritual journey?

ASSOCIATIONS OFFERING SPIRITUAL SUPPORT TO
HEALTHCARE PROFESSIONALS

Christian Support: Physicians, Dentists, Nurses,
Nurse-Midwives, Social Workers
   Christian Medical and Dental Associations (CMDA)
      www.cmdahome.org
   Christian Medical and Dental Society (CMDS) (for students)
      www.cmdahome.org
   Christians in Healthcare
      www.Christian-healthcare.org.uk
   Nurses Christian Fellowship (NCF)
      www.ivcf.org/ncf
   Christian Nurses and Midwives (CNM)
      www.cnm.org.uk
   Society for Spirituality and Social Work
      Sssw@binghamton.edu
   Islamic Support for Physicians
      Islamic Medical Association of North America
      950 75th Street, Downers Grove, IL 60516; 630-852-2122
      imana.org

Muslim Doctors and Dental Association (MDDA)
www.mdda.org.uk
The Islamic Circle of North America
P.O. Box 3174; Jamaica, NY; 718-658-1199
Dawa Information Group
8424 Naab Road, Suite 2D; Indianapolis, IN 46260; 317-872-5159

These Web sites contain valuable articles written by Dr. Shahid Athar regarding Islamic health issues.

www.islam–usa.com
www.islamfortoday.com/athar.htm

Here are some text resources for spiritual support.

For the Christian seeker:
Holy Bible
Guideposts magazine—uplifting articles; usually Christian but sometimes representing other faith traditions
Works of Henri Nouwen
Works of Philip Yancey
Works of Thomas Merton

For the Jewish seeker:
Aaron, D. (1998), *Endless Light: The Ancient Path of the Kabbalah to Love, Spiritual Growth, and Personal Power* (New York: Berkley).
Hotz, B. W. (1986), *Back to the Sources: Reading the Classic Jewish Texts* (New York: Simon and Schuster).
Schwarz, S. (2000), *Finding a Spiritual Home: How a New Generation of Jews Can Transform the American Synagogue* (San Francisco: Jossey-Bass).

For the Muslim seeker:
Dawood, N. J. (1990), trans., *The Koran* (New York: Penguin).
Ali, M. M. (1983), trans., *The Holy Quran/English/Arabic*, rev. ed., with commentary (Lahore, Pakistan: Ahamadiyya Anjuman Ishaat Islam Lahore).
Ladinsky, D. J. (1999), trans., *The Gift: Poems by Hafiz, the Great Sufi Master* (New York: Penguin-Putnam).

For the Eastern seeker:
Dalai Lama (2001), *An Open Heart: Practicing Compassion in Everyday Life*, ed. N. Vreeland (New York: Little, Brown).

Summary of Professional Affiliations and Faith Traditions (N=65)

Profession	Catholic	Nondenominational	Protestant	Buddhist	Jewish	Hindu	Sikh	Muslim	Others
Chaplains (n=5)	1		4						
Counselors (n=2)		1					1		
Health administrator (n=1)			1						
Health educator (n=1)			1						
Physicians (n=16)	4	1	3	1	2	1		4	
Occupational therapist (n=1)		1							
Psychologist (n=1)				1					
Physical therapist (n=1)			1						
Registered nurses (n=35)	7	17	10						1
Social workers (n=2)	1		1						

Endnotes

ACKNOWLEDGMENTS

1. Haas, David (1994), "We Are Called." *Gather*, 2nd ed. Copyright (c) 1988 by GIA Publications, Inc., 7404 South Mason Avenue, Chicago, IL 60638. All rights reserved.

I. SPIRITUAL CAREGIVING: HEALTHCARE AS A MINISTRY

1. Nouwen, H. (2002), *Ministry and Spirituality* (New York: Continuum), 234–235.

2. Nouwen, *Ministry and Spirituality*, 235.

3. Nouwen, *Ministry and Spirituality*, 236.

4. Mohrmann, M. E. (1995), *Medicine as Ministry: Reflections on Suffering, Ethics and Hope* (Cleveland: Pilgrim Press), 9–10.

5. Carson, V. B. (1989), *Spiritual Dimensions of Nursing Practice* (Philadelphia: W. B. Saunders), 53–54.

6. Nouwen, *Ministry and Spirituality*, 236.

7. Karaban, R. A. (1998), *Responding to God's Call: A Survival Guide* (San Jose, Calif.: Resource Publications), 15.

8. Carson, V. B., and Koenig, H. G. (2002), *Parish Nursing: Stories of Service and Care* (Philadelphia: Templeton Foundation Press), 1–2.

9. Athar, S. (2002), "Self-discovery: A Muslim Physician's Personal Journey," *Park Ridge Center Bulletin*, January/February, 9–10.

10. Turner, S. (1990), "Lean, Green, and Meaningless," *Christianity Today*, September 24, 26–27; Carson, V. (1993), "Spirituality: Generic or Christian," *Journal of Christian Nursing* 10(1): 24–27.

11. Plante, T. G., and Sherman, A. C. (2001), *Faith and Health: Psychological Perspectives* (New York: Guilford Press), 7.

12. Emmons, R. A., and Crumpler, C. A. (1999), "Religion and Spirituality: The Roles of Sanctification and the Concept of God," *International Journal for the Psychology of Religion* 9(1): 17–24.

2. THE STATE OF THE CURRENT HEALTHCARE SYSTEM

1. Benson, H. (1996), *Timeless Healing: The Power and Biology of Belief* (New York: Scribner), 97; Nouwen, H. (2002), *Ministry and Spirituality* (New York: Continuum), 234–235; Neal, J. (May 2000), "Work as Service to the Divine: Giving Our Gifts Selflessly and with Joy," *American Behavioral Scientist* 43(8): 1316–1333.

2. Dworkin, R. W. (May 2001), "Why Doctors Are Down," *Commentary*, 43–47; Schroeder, S. A. (1992), "The Troubled Profession: Is Medicine's Glass Half Full or Half Empty?" *Annals of Internal Medicine* 116: 583–592; Aiken, L. H., et al. (2002), "Hospital Nurse Staffing and Patient Mortality, Nurse Burnout, and Job Dissatisfaction," *Journal of the American Medical Association* 288: 1987–1993.

3. Eisenberg, D., and Seiger, M. (2003), "The Doctor Won't See You Now: The Soaring Cost of Malpractice Insurance Is Becoming a Worry for Everyone," *Time*, June 9, 46–60.

4. Girard, N. J. (2003), "Renewal of the Spirit," *AORN Journal* 77(3): 540–542; Severinsson, E. (2003), "Moral Stress and Burnout: Qualitative Content Analysis," *Nursing and Health Sciences* 5(1): 59–66; Culliford, L. (2002), "Spirituality and Clinical Care: Spiritual Values and Skills Are Increasingly Recognized as Necessary Aspects of Clinical Care," *British Medical Journal* 325(7378): 1434–1435; Weiner, E. L., et al. (2001), "A Qualitative Study of Physicians' Own Wellness-Promotion Practices," *Western Journal of Medicine* 174(1): 19–23.

5. Bazan, W., Dwyer, D. (1998), "Assessing Spirituality: Healthcare Organizations Must Address Their Employees' Spiritual Needs," *Health Progress* 79(2): 20–24.

6. Mitroff, I. I., and Denton, E. A. (1999), *A Spiritual Audit of Corporate America* (San Francisco: Jossey-Bass), 155, 157.

7. Mohrmann, M. E. (1995), *Medicine as Ministry: Reflections on Suffering, Ethics and Hope* (Cleveland: Pilgrim Press), 39.

8. Mitroff and Denton, *Spiritual Audit*, 85.

9. Trott, D. C. (1997), "Spiritual Well-Being of Workers: An Exploratory Study of Spirituality in the Workplace," Ph.D. dissertation, abstract in *Dissertation Abstracts International* 57(9A): 4152.

10. Mitroff and Denton, *Spiritual Audit*, 85; Trott, "Spiritual Well-Being of Workers," 4152.

11. Acker, K. (2000), "Developmental Processes and Structures Requisite to the Integration of Spirituality and Work," Ph.D. dissertation, The Fielding Graduate Institute, *Dissertation Abstracts International* 61(2-B): 1107. Mitroff and Denton, *Spiritual Audit*, 85; Trott, "Spiritual Well-Being of Workers," 4152; Wasylyshyn, K. M. (Winter 2001), "On the Full Actualization of Psychology in Business," *Consulting Psychology Journal: Practice and Research* 53(1): 10–21.

12. Mitroff and Denton, *Spiritual Audit*, 85.

13. Canda, E. R., and Furman, L. D. (1999), *Spiritual Diversity in Social Work Practice: The Heart of Helping* (New York: Free Press), 183–213.

14. Acker, "Developmental Processes and Structures," 1107.

15. Haring, B. (1982), *Healing Mission of the Church in the Coming Decades* (Washington, D.C.: Center for Applied Research in the Apostolate); O'Brien, M. E.

(1999), *Spirituality in Nursing: Standing on Holy Ground* (Sudbury, Mass.: James and Bartlett Publishers), 85–117; Sharts-Harpo, N. C. (2000), "Reality Shock in the Workplace," in *Nursing Now! Today's Issues, Tomorrow's Trends*, 2nd ed., ed. J. Catalano (Philadelphia: F. A. Davis), 347–371.

3. ENVISIONING THE IDEAL

1. Joint Commission on the Accreditation of Healthcare Organizations, "2004 Comprehensive Accreditation Manual for Hospitals: The Official Handbook" (Chicago: Joint Commission of the Accreditation of Healthcare Organizations), available online at www.jcaho.org
2. Bazan, W., and Dwyer, D. (1998), "Assessing Spirituality: Healthcare Organizations Must Address Their Employees' Spiritual Needs," *Health Progress* 79(2): 20–24.
3. Graber, D. R., and Johnson, J. A. (January–February 2001), "Spirituality and Healthcare Organizations," *Journal of Healthcare Management* 46(2): 39–50.
4. For more information about the Planetree philosophy see Highline Hospital's Web site, www.HighlineHospital.org, or call the hospital at 206-431-5247.
5. Hale, W. D., and Bennett, R. G. (2000), *Building Healthy Communities through Medical-Religious Partnerships* (Baltimore, Md.: Johns Hopkins University Press).
6. Richardt, S., and Magers, J. (November–December 1997), "Spirituality for Lay Leaders: System Program Stressed the Motivation Behind the Ministry," *Health Progress* 78(6): 18–19, 34.

4. PREPARATION FOR SPIRITUAL CAREGIVING

1. Personal communication between Dr. Harold G. Koenig and Chaplain Will Kinnaird, chair, Joint Commission for the Accreditation of Pastoral Services. Chaplain Kinnaird can be reached at National VA Chaplain Center, 757-728-3180, Will.Kinnaird@med.va.gov.
2. Koenig, H. G., McCullough, M. E., and Larson, D. B. (2001), *Handbook of Religion and Health* (New York: Oxford University Press).
3. Kleinman, A. (1987), "Anthropology and Psychiatry: The Role of Culture in Cross-Cultural Research on Illness," *British Journal of Psychiatry* 151: 447–454 and Kleinman, A. (1988), *Rethinking Psychiatry: From Cultural Category to Personal Experience* (New York: Free Press).
4. Koenig, McCullough, and Larson, *Handbook of Religion and Health*, 400, 429, 431.
5. Lannin, D. R., et al. (1998), "Influences of Socioeconomic and Cultural Factors on Racial Differences in Late-Stage Presentation of Breast Cancer." *Journal of the American Medical Association* 279: 1801–1807.
6. U.S. Constitution, Amendment XIV:1, "No State shall make or enforce any law which shall abridge the privileges or immunities of citizens of the United States." See *Cantwell v. Connecticut*, 310 U.S. 296 (1940).

7. *Jacobson v. Massachusetts*, 197 U.S. 11 (1905).

8. Exception to religious exemptions, *Kleid v. Board of Education of Fulton*, 406 F Supp. 902 (W.D. Ky. 1976).

9. Filenbaum, J. R. (Spring 2000), "Your Rights to Avoid Immunizations," *Innovations.*

10. McMullen, P. C. (1989), "Religious Belief, Legal Issues, and Health Care," in *Spiritual Dimensions of Nursing Practice*, ed. V. B. Carson (Philadelphia: W. B. Saunders), 132–146.

11. Application of the President and Directors of Georgetown College, Inc., 331 F. Z. A. 1000 (D.C. Cir. 1964).

12. *In re* Estate of Brooks, 32 III. 2d 361, 205 N.E. 2nd 435 (1965).

13. Robinson, B. A. (2002), "Faith Healing: Legal Aspects," www. religioustolerance.org/medical1.htm.

14. "No Cure for Cancer: Tennessee Mom, Preacher Accused of Letting Girl Die by Turning to God," ABCNews.com, October 3, 2002, www.abcnews.go.com/sections/us/DailyNews/religious_defense021003.html.

15. Asser, S. M., and Swan, R. (1998), "Child Fatalities from Religion-Motivated Medical Neglect," *Pediatrics* 101(4): 625–629.

16. Robinson, B. A., "Faith Healing."

17. Falwell, J., "Your Faith Stops Here," WorldNetDaily, February 22, 2003, www.worldnetdaily.com/news/article.asp?ARTICLE_ID=31180.

18. Kasdan, I. (1998), Agudath Israel of America National Public Policy Position Paper: I. Religious and Civil Rights, www.jlaw.com/LawPolicy/OU2.html.

19. Bellos, A. (2001), "Can Religion Trump the Bioethics Debate?" www.emory.edu/college/HYBRIDVIGOR/issue4/religion.htm.

20. Darryl Macer (1998), "Bioethics Is Love of Life: An Alternative Textbook," www.biol.tsukuba.ac.jp/~macer/BLL.html.

5. PROVIDING SPIRITUAL CARE

1. Mohrmann, M. E. (1995), *Medicine as Ministry: Reflections on Suffering, Ethics, and Hope* (Cleveland: Pilgrim Press), 109–111.

2. Shelly, J. A. (2000), *Spiritual Care: A Guide for Caregivers* (Downers Grove, Ill.: InterVarsity Press), 39–40.

3. King, D. (2000), *Faith, Spirituality, and Medicine* (New York: Haworth Press), 54.

4. King, *Faith, Spirituality, and Medicine*, 54.

5. Ehman, J., et al. (1999), "Do Patients Want Physicians to Inquire About Their Spiritual or Religious Beliefs If They Become Gravely Ill?" *Archives of Internal Medicine* 159: 1803–1806 and Silvestri, G. A., et al. (2003), "Importance of Faith on Medical Decisions Regarding Cancer Care," *Journal of Clinical Oncology* 21: 1379–1382.

6. Koenig, H. G. (2002), *Spirituality in Patient Care* (Philadelphia: Templeton Foundation Press), 13–15.

7. Ehman, "Do Patients Want Physicians to Inquire?"

8. Silvestri, "Importance of Faith."

9. Koenig, *Spirituality in Patient Care*, 7–8.

10. Shelly, *Spiritual Care*, 30.

11. Koenig, *Spirituality in Patient Care*, 21.

12. Koenig, H. G., et al. (1991), "Religious Perspectives of Doctors, Nurses, Patients, and Families," *Journal of Pastoral Care* 45(3): 254–267.

13. Iowa Intervention Project (2000), Nursing Interventions Classification, 3rd ed., ed. J. C. McCloskey and G. M. Bulechek (St. Louis, Mo.: Mosby).

14. Iowa Outcomes Project (2000), Nursing Outcomes Classification, 2nd ed., ed. M. Johnson and S. Moorhead (St. Louis, Mo.: Mosby), www.nursing.uiowa.edu/centers/cncce/noc.

15. Carson, V. B. (1989), *Spiritual Dimensions of Nursing Practice* (Philadelphia: W. B. Saunders), 157.

16. Carson, *Spiritual Dimensions of Nursing Practice*, 158.

17. Carson, *Spiritual Dimensions of Nursing Practice*, 159.

18. Shelly, *Spiritual Care*, 75.

19. Shelly, *Spiritual Care*, 75–86.

20. Lewis, C. S. (1985), "Prayer," in *Modern Spirituality: An Anthology*, ed. J. Garvey (Springfield, Ill.: Templegate Publishers).

21. Pargament, K. L., et al. (2001), "Religious Struggle As a Predictor of Mortality among Medically Ill Elderly Patients: A Two-Year Longitudinal Study," *Archives of Internal Medicine* 161: 1881–1885.

22. Athar, S. (2002), "Self-Discovery: A Muslim Physician's Personal Journey," *The Park Ridge Center Bulletin*, January/February, 10.

6. GIVING SPIRITUAL CARE: THE PATIENT WITH CHRONIC ILLNESS AND PAIN

1. Stoll, R. I. (1989), "Spirituality in Chronic Illness," in *Spiritual Dimensions of Nursing Practice*, ed. V. B. Carson (Philadelphia: W. B. Saunders), 180–216.

2. Engle, G. L. (1964), "Grief and Grieving," *American Journal of Nursing* 64: 93–98.

3. Crate, M. A. (1965), "Nursing Functions in Adaptation to Chronic Illness," *American Journal of Nursing* 65: 72–76.

4. Feldman, D. J. (1974), "Chronic Disabling Illness: A Holistic View," *Journal of Chronic Diseases* 27: 290.

5. Stoll, "Spirituality in Chronic Illness," 194.

6. Koenig, H.G., et al. (1998), "Religiosity and Remission from Depression in Medically Ill Older Patients," *American Journal of Psychiatry* 155: 536–542.

7. Stoll, "Spirituality in Chronic Illness," 194.

8. Stoll, "Spirituality in Chronic Illness," 195.

9. Psalm 23. *The NIV Quiet Time Bible: New Testament and Psalms* (Downers Grove, Ill.: InterVarsity Press, 1994), 471.

10. Koenig, H. G., (1998), "Religious Beliefs and Practices of Hospitalized

Medically Ill Older Adults," *International Journal of Geriatric Psychiatry* 13: 213–224.

11. Stedman, R. C. (1976), "Lessons from Pain," *His* 37(1): 4.

12. Benson, Herbert (1984), *Beyond the Relaxation Response* (New York: Times Books), 5–6, 106–111.

13. Benson, *Beyond the Relaxation Response*, 104.

14. Starck, R. (1983), "The Meaning of Suffering Experiences as Perceived by Hospital Clients," final report (Troy, Ala.: Troy State University School of Nursing).

15. Stoll, "Spirituality in Chronic Illness," 199.

16. Wheeler, E. G., and Dace-Lombard, J. (1989), *Living Creatively with Chronic Illness* (Ventura, Calif.: Pathfinder Publishing), 7–9.

17. Smyth, J., et al. (1999), "Effects of Writing about Stressful Experiences on Symptom Reduction with Asthma or Rheumatoid Arthritis: A Randomized Trial," *Journal of the American Medical Association* 281(14): 1304–1309.

18. U.S. Department of Health and Human Services (2002), http://aspe.hhs.gov/health/reports/physicalactivity.

19. Murray, C. (1996), *Global Burden of Disease* (Cambridge, Mass.: Harvard University Press).

7. GIVING SPIRITUAL CARE: THE DYING PATIENT

1. Jacik, M. (1989), "Spiritual Care of the Dying Adult," in *Spiritual Dimensions of Nursing Practice*, ed. V. B. Carson (Philadelphia: W. B. Saunders), 270–274.

2. Kaldjian, L., et al. (1998), "End of Life Decisions in HIV Positive Patients: The Role of Spiritual Beliefs," *AIDS* 12(1): 103–107.

3. George H. Gallup International Institute (October 1997), "Spiritual Beliefs and the Dying Process: A Report on a National Survey." Nathan Cummings Foundation and Fetzer Institute.

4. Bernardin, J. (1996), *The Journey to Peace: Reflections on Faith, Embracing Suffering, and Finding New Life* (New York: Doubleday), 1–20.

5. Jacik, "Spiritual Care of the Dying Adult."

6. Koenig, H. G. (2002), *Spirituality in Patient Care: Why, How, When, and What* (Philadelphia: Templeton Foundation Press), 7.

7. Carson, V. B. (1997), "Spiritual Care: The Needs of the Caregiver," *Seminars in Oncology Nursing* 13(4): 271–274.

8. Carson, "Spiritual Care."

9. Carson, "Spiritual Care."

10. Jacik, "Spiritual Care of the Dying Adult."

11. Walsh, K. King, M.; Jones, L. Tookman, A. Blizard, R. (2002), "Spiritual Beliefs May Affect Outcome of Bereavement: Prospective Study," *British Medical Journal*, 324(7353), June, 1551.

12. Jacik, "Spiritual Care of the Dying Adult."

8. SPIRITUAL CARE FOR SPECIAL POPULATIONS

1. Mohrmann, M. E. (1995), *Medicine as Ministry: Reflections on Suffering, Ethics, and Hope* (Cleveland: Pilgrim Press), 74.

2. Tibesar, L. J. (1986), "Pastoral Care: Helping Patients on an Inward Journey," *Health Progress* 67(4): 41–47.

3. Kayal, P. M. (1985), "Morals, Medicine, and the AIDS Epidemic," *Journal of Religion and Health* 24(3): 218.

4. Kübler-Ross, E. (1987), *AIDS: The Ultimate Challenge* (New York: MacMillan), 13.

5. Murphy, P. (March–April 1986), "Pastoral Care and Persons with AIDS," *American Journal of Hospice Care*, 39.

6. Tibesar, "Pastoral Care," 45; O'Neill, D. P., and Kenny, E. K. (1998), "Spirituality and Chronic Illness," *Image—The Journal of Nursing Scholarship* 30:275–280.

7. Koenig, H. G. et al. (2001), *Handbook of Religion and Health* (New York: Oxford University Press), 97–101.

8. Koenig, *Handbook*.

9. Sabbagh, M. N. (2003), "Alzheimer's Disease Diagnosis and Treatment: Past, Present, and Future," presentation given in Phoenix, Arizona, at the 12th Annual Caregiver Conference, Visions of Hope: Living Today, Planning Tomorrow, March 21, 2003.

10. Buckwalter, G. (2003), "Addressing the Spiritual and Religious Needs of Persons with Profound Memory Loss," *Home Healthcare Nurse* 21(1): 20–21.

11. King, D. (2000), *Faith, Spirituality, and Medicine: Toward the Making of the Healing Practitioner* (New York: Haworth Pastoral Press), 93.

12. Saudia, T. L., et al. (1991), "Health, Locus of Control, and Helpfulness of Prayer," *Heart and Lung* 20(1): 60–65.

13. Harris, R. C., et al. (1995), "The Role of Religion in Heart-Transplant Recipients' Long-Term Health and Well-Being," *Journal of Religion and Health* 34(1): 17–32.

14. Florell, J. L. (1973), "Crisis-Intervention in Orthopedic Surgery: Empirical Evidence of the Effectiveness of a Chaplain Working with Surgery Patients," *Bulletin of the Professional Hospital Association* 37(2): 29–36.

9. NURTURING THE SELF: NURTURING THE SPIRIT

1. Mohrmann, M. E. (1995), *Medicine as Ministry: Reflections on Suffering, Ethics, and Hope* (Cleveland: Pilgrim Press), 109–117.

2. Mohrmann, *Medicine as Ministry*, 34–50.

3. Mohrmann, *Medicine as Ministry*, 50.

4. Jourard, S. M. (1976), *Transparent Self: Self Disclosure and Well-Being* (New York: Wiley).

5. Stoll, R.I. (1989), "The Essence of Spirituality," in *Spiritual Dimensions of Nursing Practice,* ed. V. B. Carson (Philadelphia: W. B. Saunders), 6.

6. Nouwen, H. (1993), *Life of the Beloved: Spiritual Living in a Secular World* (New York: Crossroad Publishing), 9–21.

7. Nouwen, *Life of the Beloved*, 18.

8. Nouwen, *Life of the Beloved*, 30–31.

9. "I Spend Time in Worship or Prayer Every Day," www.gallup.com /subscription/?m=f&c_id=11449.

10. Koenig, H. G., et al. (1991), "Religious Perspective of Doctors, Nurses, Patients, and Families: Some Interesting Differences," *Journal of Pastoral Care* 45: 254–267.

11. Schoenberger, N. E., et al. (2002), "Opinions and Practices of Medical Rehabilitation Professionals Regarding Prayer and Meditation," *Journal of Alternative and Complementary Medicine* 8(1): 59–69.

12. Marsh, V., Beard, M., and Adams, B. (1999), "Job Stress and Burnout: The Mediational Effect of Spiritual Well-Being and Hardiness among Nurses," *Journal of Theory Construction and Testing* 3: 13–19.

13. Taylor, A. G., et al. (1998), "ED Staff Members' Personal Use of Complementary Therapies and Their Recommendations to ED Patients: A Southeastern US Regional Survey," *Journal of Emergency Nursing* 24(6): 495–499.

10. A DAVID–AND–GOLIATH MATCH:
TAKING ON THE SYSTEM

1. Propst, L. R., et al. (1992), "Comparative Efficacy of Religions and Nonreligious Cognitive-Behavior Therapy for the Treatment of Clinical Depression in Religious Individuals," *Journal of Consulting and Clinical Psychology* 60: 94–103.

2. De Saint-Exupery, A. (1943), *The Little Prince* (New York: Harcourt).

APPENDIX A: RELIGIOUS BELIEFS AND PRACTICES

1. Carson, V. B. (1989), *Spiritual Dimensions of Nursing Practice* (Philadelphia: W. B. Saunders), 80–81, 85–86, 90–92, 95–96, 100–102.

2. Griffith, K. J. (1996), *The Religious Aspects of Nursing Care*, Box 72072, 4479 W. Tenth Avenue, Vancouver, B.C., Canada V6R 4P2.

APPENDIX B: SPIRITUAL ASSESSMENT RESOURCES

1. Used with permission from Puchalski, C. M., and Romer, A. L. (2000), "Taking a Spiritual History Allows Clinicians to Understand Patients More Fully," *Journal of Palliative Medicine* 3: 129–137. Web site: www.gwish.org/id69.htm.

2. Koenig, H. G. (2002), "An 83-Year-Old Woman with Chronic Illness and Strong Religious Beliefs," *Journal of the American Medical Association* 288(4): 487–493.

3. Matthews, D. A., and Clark, C. (1998), *The Faith Factor* (New York: Viking).

4. Maugans, T. A. (1996), "The SPIRITual History," *Archives of Family Medicine* 5: 11–16.

5. Anandarajah, G., and Hight, E. (2001), "Spirituality and Medical Practice: Using HOPE Questions as a Practical Tool for Spiritual Assessment," *American Family Physician* 63(1): 81–88.

6. Lo, B., Quill, T., and Tulsky, J. (1999), "Discussing Palliative Care with Patients," *Annals of Internal Medicine* 130: 744–749.

APPENDIX C: RESOURCES FOR SPIRITUAL SUPPORT
AND NURTURE

1. Dr. Leslie Van Dover and Diane Bergman, McMaster University, 1993.

2. Patterson, R. B. "Writing Your Spiritual Autobiography: Pathway to a Stronger Faith," *Liguorian* 91(1): 22–23.

Contributors

The following list represents the many professionals who generously shared their time and stories with us to make this book a reality. We thank them.

Eileen Altenhofer, R.N., parish nurse, Seattle, Wash.

Dr. Shahid Athar, endocrinologist, Indianapolis, Ind.

Dr. Tarif Bakdash, Syria.

Dr. Don C. Berry, principal founder and president, Institute of Religion and Health, Charleston, S.C., and Augusta, Ga., www.instituteofreligionandhealth.com and www.faithandhealthmatters.com.

Dr. Shyam Bhat, psychiatrist, Springfield, Ill.

Jay Brashear, occupational therapist for Tender Loving Care–Staff Builders, Phoenix, Ariz.

Dr. Herman Brecher, internal medicine, Seton Medical Group, Catonsville, Md.

Dee Brooks, R.N., pediatrics, Milton, Vt.

Sandra E. Brown, family nurse practitioner; currently a doctoral student focusing on spiritual issues, Miami, Fla.

Marilyn Bullock, R.N., long-term care, Boston, Mass.

Dr. Patricia Camp, parish nurse coordinator, Barlow, Ky.

Dr. Kong Chhean, clinical psychologist, Long Beach Asian Pacific Mental Health Program, Department of Mental Health, Los Angeles County, Calif.

Dr. Gunnar E. Christiansen, retired ophthalmologist, currently a volunteer for the National Alliance for the Mentally Ill, Santa Ana, Calif.

Harriet Coeling, nursing faculty, Kent State University, Kent, Ohio.

Dr. Sagrid Eleanor Edman, retired dean, Bethel College, St. Paul, Minn.

Susan Feldman, a Masters-prepared nurse; currently working in health care sales and marketing, Baltimore, Md.

Chaplain Jeffrey Flowers, director of pastoral care, Medical College of Georgia, Augusta, Ga.

Genie Ford, pediatrics nurse, adjunct professor of nursing science for an Associate of Arts program, full-time MSN student, Edmund, Okla.

Vicki Germer, psychiatric nurse, clinical specialist and reflexologist, Jacksonville, Tex.

Dr. Thomas Grace, plastic and reconstructive surgeon, Baltimore, Md.

Dr. Jack Hasson, Birmingham, Ala.

Shirley Herron, BScN, retired nurse, spiritual director, consultant in palliative care, Etobicoke, Ontario, Canada.

Nancy Hines, R.N., Rochester, N.Y.

Kay Hurd, manager, Congregational Health Ministries and Healthy Congregations at Somerset Medical Center, Somerville, N.J.

Miriam Jacik, retired R.N., oncology specialist, pastoral care counselor; currently runs a bereavement support group for her parish in Greenbelt, Md.

Dr. Sandra Jamison, retired nursing professor, currently director, Nurses Christian Fellowship Faculty and Graduate Student Ministry, Dillsburg, Pa.

Charity Johansson, Ph.D., physical therapist, Elon University, Elon, North Carolina.

Dr. Dharma Singh Khalsa, anesthesiologist, Tucson, Ariz.

Joyce Kinstlinger, community resource counselor, Northfield, Vt.

Charmin Koenig, former X-ray technician, nurse; now full-time mother and wife, Durham, N.C.

Carole Kornelis, parish nurse, Lynden, Wash.

Othelia Lee, social work professor, North Carolina State University, Raleigh, N.C.

Catherine Lick, parish nurse, Troy, Mich.

Dr. Alton L. Lightsey, retired pediatric oncologist; involved in a faith clinic in a church in Evans, Ga.

Martha Loveland, R.N., healthcare administrator of a holistic health clinic, Helena, Mont.

Karen McCauley, R.N., homecare, Baltimore, Md.

Florika Miranda, R.N., account executive for Tender Loving Care–Staff Builders, Amherst, N.Y.

Diane Molitor, R.N., Ellicott City, Md.

Reverend Rodger Murchison, associate pastor, First Baptist Church, Augusta, Ga.

Dr. Daniel Ober, hospice medical director, Milford, N.H.

Elizabeth Page, R.N., Kingston, N.H.

Dr. Michael W. Parker, specialty in gerontology from a social work and psychology perspective, University of Alabama, Tuscaloosa, Ala.

Dr. Jirpesh R. Patel, child psychiatrist, Duke Medical Center, Durham, N.C.

Amy Pollman, psychiatric home care nurse, Tender Loving Care Home Health Services, Phoenix, Ariz.

Cynthia Ann Poort, R.N., director, mental health program, Visiting Nurses Association, Grand Rapids, Mich.

Sister Karen Pozniak, SND. de N., NACC Cert., Catholic sister, educator, chaplain.

Kelly Preston, R.N., formerly congregational health program coordinator for the Ingalls Center of Pastoral Ministries, Baptist Health System of Alabama, Birmingham, Ala.

Dr. Christina Puchalski, founder and director of the George Washington University Institute for Spirituality and Health, Washington, D.C.

Carole Richards, pediatric nurse, St. George, Vt.

Beatrice Rosen, R.N., St. George, Vt.

Ada Scharf, R.N., Nurse Christian Fellowship staff member, Olean, N.Y.

Margie Schmier, homecare nurse, Baltimore, Md.

Dr. Franz Sewchand, internist, Seton Medical Group, Catonsville, Md.

Dr. Hasan Shanawani, Durham, N.C.

Nancy Shoemaker, psychiatric nurse, clinical specialist, Baltimore, Md.

Dr. T. D. Singh, chemist, counselor, educator, Bhaktivedanta Institute and Vedanta and Science Educational Research Foundation, Calcutta, India.

Chaplain Robb Small, director of pastoral care/chaplain, Fort Payne, Ala.

Dianne Smith, pediatrics nurse, Westford, Vt.

Joanne Smith, R.N., administrator, Boston, Mass.

Dr. Karen Soeken, nursing professor, University of Maryland School of Nursing, Baltimore, Md.

Dr. Julie Steiner, internist, Seton Medical Group, Catonsville, Md.

Carol Story, director, Puget Sound Parish Nurse Ministries, Everett, Wash.

Dr. Bernita Taylor, family practice, Seton Medical Group, Catonsville, Md.

Brenda Thornton, R.N., account executive in home care for Tender Loving Care–Staff Builders, Amherst, N.Y.

Evelyn Yapp, psychiatric nurse, clinical specialist, Baltimore, Md.

Index